DIABETES

The Essential Guide

Need
— 2 —
Know

Sue
Marshall

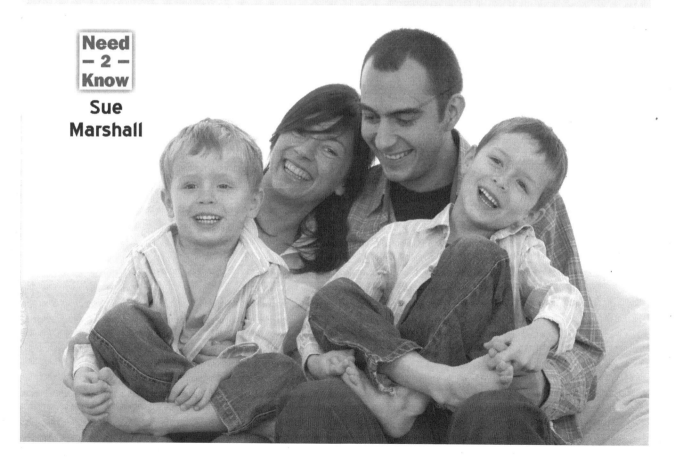

First published in Great Britain in 2008 by
Need2Know
Remus House
Coltsfoot Drive
Peterborough
PE2 9JX
Telephone 01733 898103
Fax 01733 313524
www.need2knowbooks.co.uk

Need2Know is an imprint of Forward Press Ltd.
www.forwardpress.co.uk
SB ISBN 978-1-86144-059-4
Cover photograph: Stock Xpert

Contents

Introduction

Rates of diagnoses of diabetes are sky-rocketing across the globe, and it's becoming a growing concern to governments who have to fund the cost of health services.

There are currently at least 2 million people with diabetes in the UK, but it's believed that about 1 million people may have diabetes and not know it. Of the 2 million diagnosed diabetics, approximately 25% have Type 1 diabetes and the rest have Type 2.

Type 2 was once seen as a disease of adults. Today, this type of diabetes is also growing at alarming rates in children and adolescents. In the US, it is estimated that Type 2 diabetes represents between eight and 45% of new-onset diabetes cases in children, depending on geographic location. Over a 20-year period, Type 2 diabetes has doubled in children from Japan so that it is now more common than Type 1. In native and aboriginal children in North America and Australia, the prevalence rate of Type 2 diabetes ranges from 1.3% to 5.3%.

Diabetes is not a disease – you cannot catch it, you develop it. The factors that trigger this development vary, but there are two main causes which separate the two most commonly occurring forms of the condition; Type 1 (insulin dependent) and Type 2 (non-insulin dependent). Both types can be treated with insulin, but those with Type 2 do produce some of their own insulin.

Packed with practical advice and the latest medical information, this book is here to help. Its easy-to-read style looks at what the diabetic condition is, how a person becomes diabetic, the types of treatment available and how to live a healthy, happy life with the condition. A glossary of key terms is included at the back of the book.

With some good advice, some understanding of what you're eating and the effect it has on your blood sugars, as well as a healthy dose of discipline, you can find a balance between having a chronic condition and having a life.

Whether you have just been diagnosed with diabetes, or work, teach or live with someone who has the condition, this book will arm you with all the essential facts you need to know.

Disclaimer

This book is for general information about diabetes. It is not intended to replace professional medical advice. It can be used alongside medical advice, but anyone with concerns about their diabetes is strongly advised to consult their healthcare professional.

Whilst every care has been taken to validate the contents of this guide up to the time of going to press, the author advises that she does not claim medical qualifications. The reader should seek advice from a qualified medical practitioner before undertaking any particular course of treatment.

Chapter One

Symptoms, Diagnosis and Types

What is diabetes?

Diabetes is the inability of your body to control your blood sugar level on its own. A doctor will diagnose you with diabetes if your blood sugar reading is too high – usually this is more than eight millomoles per litre (mmols/L).

Symptoms

The main symptoms of diabetes are:

- Increased thirst.
- Needing to urinate unusually often – especially at night.
- Extreme tiredness.
- Weight loss.
- Blurred vision.

There are two types of diabetes – Type 1 and Type 2. Type 1 diabetes develops much more quickly, usually over a few weeks, and symptoms are normally very obvious.

Type 2 diabetes develops more slowly and the symptoms are usually less severe. Some people may not notice any symptoms at all and their diabetes is only picked up in a routine medical check-up. In other cases, people may put the symptoms down to getting older or overworking.

In both types of diabetes the symptoms are quickly relieved once the diabetes is treated. Early treatment will also reduce the chances of developing serious health problems.

What happens in non-diabetics?

In non-diabetics, blood sugar is controlled via a feedback mechanism, which works like this:

- Food is eaten.
- Blood sugar rises as food is digested.
- Blood goes to the pituitary gland in the brain, which assesses the blood sugar level.
- If the level is too high, the pituitary gland releases a 'messenger' that travels in the blood and tells the pancreas to release insulin.
- The insulin brings down the blood sugar level.
- If the blood sugar level is too low, the pituitary gland releases a 'messenger' that tells the liver to release energy in the form of glucagon. This then raises the blood sugar level.

By releasing these messengers, the pituitary reacts to the blood sugar level until it is balanced. This explains why it's known as a feedback mechanism.

What happens in a diabetic?

Type 1 diabetes

If you're diagnosed with Type 1 diabetes it means you have a genetic component whereby you can't produce any of your own insulin. Historically, all childhood diabetes has been Type 1.

Some children are given only one type of insulin, whereas others may have two. They have one or two injections a day, sometimes more. See chapter 7 for further information on how insulin treatment profiles may change as children grow.

Type 1 diabetes is caused by the body's immune system mistaking the insulin producing beta cells (located in the islets of Langerhans in the pancreas) as something alien and destroying them. Currently there is no way to predict who will develop this type of diabetes, but if any of your ancestors had it you stand a chance of developing it.

Developing Type 1 diabetes has nothing whatsoever to do with having had a bad diet. The link between Type 1 diabetes and diet is that you will now be able to feel how different foods affect you – something very sugary will have a distinct and definite effect. If you have just been diagnosed with diabetes, you will have to do blood tests and judge your food (mainly by 'counting carbohydrates') so that you can give yourself the right dose of insulin (by injection or insulin pump) to balance out the food eaten.

You must also remember that your body needs insulin to survive. If you go off your food, you cannot stop taking your insulin as you will become very unwell. So if you plan on losing weight by reducing what you eat, don't make the mistake of thinking you won't need insulin. If you want to lose weight, reduce your insulin to match your reduced intake of food, but don't stop taking your medication.

Working out dosages

If you've got Type 1 diabetes, you will have to do a blood test in order to assess your blood sugar level. It's then a case of doing the maths to figure out what dose is needed.

The maths is:

- Your blood sugar level (it's best to do a blood test prior to a meal).
- The food you are about to eat.
- What you are about to do after your meal and how energetic it is.

'If you go off your food, you cannot stop taking your insulin as you will become very unwell. So if you plan on losing weight by reducing what you eat, don't make the mistake of thinking you won't need insulin.'

There isn't a specific calculation for this as everyone is different and, given a bit of time, you'll get used to judging the right dose, but it takes practice, persistence and continual monitoring of blood sugars. You won't always get ideal blood test results, but you will learn how your body reacts to the food and insulin you give it.

The simplest guideline (and it is only a guideline) is one unit of insulin for every 10g of carbohydrate. In some places, 10g of carbohydrate is also known as 'one exchange', which makes one unit of insulin for one carbohydrate exchange.

The amount of insulin you give yourself will be based on:

- The type of insulin it is and how it works.

- Your body size (we're all different and how much insulin we need varies accordingly).

- What you are about to eat (mainly according to the carbohydrates in the dish).

- What you are about to do (if you finish your lunch and are going to do something energetic, you will need less insulin than if you're doing something unenergetic).

Counting carbohydrates is probably the thing that is newest to people who are diagnosed with diabetes – it takes some getting used to, but you will get the hang of it after a while. In many ways, it's similar to counting calories just as you would on a diet.

We'll look into counting carbohydrates in more detail later on in chapter 5.

Type 2 diabetes

If you are diagnosed with Type 2 diabetes it means that you can make your own insulin, but its effectiveness is compromised.

Type 2 diabetes is associated with bad diet, lack of exercise and generally having too much weight. There are some medical conditions and genetic factors (e.g. the 'fat gene') which indicate that such weight gain is down to certain metabolic factors, but about 80% of Type 2 diabetes is down to 'less than ideal' eating habits and excess weight.

When you are first diagnosed as having Type 2 diabetes, you are likely to have your diet reviewed and you may be put on pills to stabilise your blood sugar levels. It's unlikely that you will be put on insulin, at least not initially, but that may come later.

It appears that changes in society such as the increased access to highly-processed carbohydrates, as found in fast foods, and the greater choice we now have in supermarkets, which we tend to drive and not walk to, may have led to Type 2 becoming an 'epidemic' of our times.

Metabolic Syndrome

Type 2 diabetes is sometimes associated with Metabolic Syndrome. Metabolic Syndrome is also known as Metabolic Syndrome X, Syndrome X, Insulin Resistance Syndrome, Reaven's Syndrome or CHAOS (Australia).

What is it?

This syndrome is characterised by a group of metabolic risk factors in one person. The dominant risk factors for this syndrome appear to be abdominal obesity and insulin resistance. Other characteristics associated with the syndrome include physical inactivity, premature aging and hormonal imbalance. There may also be a genetic predisposition involved in developing it – if your parents had it then you are more likely to develop it. Other factors such as excess body fat and physical inactivity can contribute towards insulin resistance and Metabolic Syndrome in these people.

The American Heart Association and the National Heart, Lung and Blood Institute recommend that this syndrome should be identified by the presence of three or more of these components:

1. **Waist circumference:** men – equal to or greater than 40 inches (102 cm); women – equal to or greater than 35 inches (88 cm).

2. **Triglycerides (or cholesterol levels):** equal to or greater than 150 mg/dL; Reduced HDL (good) cholesterol: men – less than 40 mg/dL; women – less than 50 mg/dL.

3. **Blood pressure:** equal to or greater than 130/85 mm Hg.

4. **Fasting glucose** (a blood glucose test taken at least eight hours after you last ate – usually first thing in the morning, before breakfast): equal to or greater than 10 mmols/L.

The cause of the syndrome is unknown – it appears to be complex, although most patients are older, obese, don't move around much and have a degree of insulin resistance. There is debate regarding whether obesity or insulin resistance is the cause of the syndrome or if they are consequences of a more far-reaching metabolic derangement (high weight, high cholesterol, high blood pressure, high blood sugar).

There is some research that seems to show that certain individuals do not know when they are full and therefore overeat. Their bodies do not register that they have had enough, causing obesity. But engaging in good practice about food (eat healthy foods, monitor your portion sizes and frequency of eating) will help prevent weight gain and aid weight loss. Parents need to oversee this from the start so children learn the discipline not to overeat just because food is available.

Other forms of diabetes

Maturity Onset Diabetes of the Young (MODY)

This is a rare form of diabetes that is caused by a mistake in a single gene. Six types of MODY (caused by six different genes) have been identified and are diagnosed by genetic tests. It's often diagnosed simply as Type 1 diabetes in very young children, most being under the age of one. With appropriate diagnosis some of these children have later come off mainstream diabetes drugs (insulin in particular).

Brittle diabetes

This term is applied to people who have diabetes that is very hard to control. It is characterised by sudden, dramatic hypos (where the blood sugar drops too low) that come on without warning and can mean that you become unconscious. There is a screening process for brittle diabetes which you (or your doctor) can request.

Diabetes – family, friends, colleagues and teachers

The diagnosis of diabetes can have a huge impact on you, but it can also affect those around you, particularly at home. Type 1 diabetes is arguably a more serious condition – without the insulin injections you can get into trouble quite quickly (possibly resulting in a 'diabetic coma' or becoming unconscious).

Family

It's lonely enough when learning to live with a medical condition – it can occupy a lot of your thoughts at the start. Having your family on board while you get used to living with diabetes can be a huge help.

Much of handling diabetes well comes down to eating good food. You may need to take a long hard look at your diet and the diet of your family. If your diet improves then theirs can too, which can only be to their benefit.

Friends

More and more people are being diagnosed with diabetes. There are now an estimated 2 million people with the condition in the UK, of which about 25% have Type 1 diabetes – so you're not alone!

'The diagnosis of diabetes can have a huge impact on you, but it can also affect those around you, particularly at home.'

With Type 1 you need to do blood tests and injections that might draw attention to you. However, the longer you have diabetes, the less self-conscious you become. I used to hide in the toilet to do a blood test and injection. Now I'll happily do a blood test while standing in a queue waiting for a bus.

It should be easy enough to tell old friends about your diagnosis, but it may take a while before you feel you ought to share this information about yourself with new friends. Yet, they may simply figure it out when you do a blood test at some point while out with them – you should not let embarrassment stop you from doing blood tests.

When telling someone for the first time that I have diabetes, I just say something like, 'I'm diabetic. It's under control most of the time. I do injections (or take tablets, or use an insulin pump) and I might get a low blood sugar, but I keep my blood test machine handy so I should be able to tell if I'm going hypo. If I am, I've got some sugar with me and I should be fine. I'll let you know if I'm having a problem. I might need five minutes to recover if I do have a hypo.' There are more hypo tips later in the book on page 43.

You'll enjoy yourself more if you feel safe in the knowledge that others know and understand your condition and can help you should you need it.

Work

If you have either type of diabetes, you might also need the help and support of your colleagues.

For some jobs, there are legal restrictions. Check with Diabetes UK (www. diabetes.org.uk) if you have any concerns; they should be able to give you guidance on your rights and your employer's legal requirements.

Most of us don't want to impose on people and would like to keep our health to ourselves, but it's a good idea to let others know what you're dealing with. Maybe you could give them a little explanation of what diabetes is and how it might affect you on a day-to-day basis. I've always told an employer – there's a place on any job application form where you have to mention medical conditions. If you're a Type 1 diabetic you should have a blood test machine handy at all times, just in case you need to get it out and do a test.

Hypoglycaemias (where the blood sugar level drops too low), or hypos as they are more commonly known, are the main thing you'll need to inform others about. Many people have some awareness of diabetes but you may need to let them know how to help you if you have a hypo. Most diabetics know how to handle their own hypos – telling others is only a back-up should anything go wrong. See chapter 4 for more information on this.

Your colleagues at work will get used to you doing blood tests (with any luck they'll nag you if they don't see you doing them!), taking your medication and taking care over what you eat.

Diabetes and the workplace – an employer's perspective

If you are reading this as an employer, you may be interested to know that the Department of Health states that 21% of the population is clinically obese, costing more than £2 billion per year due to lost productivity (18 million days of sickness absence – UK National Audit Office). It is probable that 4% of your workforce is likely to have diabetes.

Advice and tips

- You should expect that a person applying for a job will put diabetes down on their application form if they have the condition.

- You should not consider diabetes as a reason not to employ someone.

- You should talk to your employee to see what they see as the impact of their condition on their ability to do the job. It's likely that they will just need to do blood tests from time to time and may need to have a snack in the office to raise their blood sugar.

- If they have a hypo, they may not see the need to tell you and you may not need to know about it. However, it might take 15 minutes or so for someone to recover from a hypo so let them have time out to regain their composure.

- If they do look like they need help, offer it. It might be helpful to know where they stash some sugar in case of a hypo.

'Your colleagues at work will get used to you doing blood tests (with any luck they'll nag you if they don't see you doing them!), taking your medication and taking care over what you eat.'

School and college

If you are the parent of a child with diabetes, you will need to fully inform your child's teachers. They need to know how to help your child, how to assess if they are having a hypo and how to deal with it.

While there are some children with Type 2, most children with diabetes have Type 1. It's possible that your child isn't the first one in his or her school to have diabetes so chances are the teachers will have dealt with it before. See chapter 7 for more information on childhood diabetes.

Of course, the most important part is to coach your child to look after themselves. Childhood diabetes is often more stable than diabetes through the teens when hormones start to kick-in, affecting not only blood sugar levels but behaviour and attitude, as well as having an impact on how medications can work.

Make sure they are prepared for school or college by having diabetes management equipment handy all day (and night, if necessary). They should have their blood test machine and, if required, their insulin kit.

'Make sure they are prepared for school or college by having diabetes management equipment handy all day (and night, if necessary). They should have their blood test machine and, if required, their insulin kit.'

Most children do not have to do injections during the day – they can be administered before and after school. Going on to do more injections is likely to happen later, depending on the age of your child. This is not a bad thing – it will only happen if it helps to give them better control, reflecting the needs of their more adult bodies and giving a bit more freedom regarding when and how they eat. However, they are likely to have to live with this for the rest of their lives, so the sooner they get used to it as a part of their lives, the better. Yes, it makes them different from the others, but not so very different. It does mean they have to be a bit more responsible and mature, at least about their diabetes.

If your child is going to college or university, then they're young adults and should have a good grip on their diabetes if they've had it a while.

They should:

- Let their new friends and housemates know.

- Register with a local doctor and check out what medical support is available.

- Carry their blood test and insulin injection kit with them.

- Try not to burn the candle at both ends too often!

Various organisations have packs available that will give you information on what the school needs to know and what you need to do. Contact one or all of the following for information: Diabetes UK, Juvenile Diabetes Research Foundation (JDRF), Diabetes Research and Wellness Foundation (DRWF) and the Insulin Dependent Diabetes Trust (IDDT) (see the help list at the end of the book for contact details).

Summing Up

- Your life will change with diabetes, but it needn't be dramatic. Keeping others informed will make things easier for you in the short-term and the long-term. After a while you won't think anything of telling someone else. It's just part of your life.

- Get as much information as you can about the type of diabetes you think you have, but take the time to read it slowly. It might be a lot of information, so allow some time for it to sink in.

- Start to look at the way your body reacts to certain food types (including liquids).

- Get used to blood testing – these days it's really not that big of a chore but you need to help yourself get into the habit of doing them.

- Taking more exercise is good for all of us, not just those who may need to lose weight. Try to incorporate more into each day – remember that stairs are your friends!

Chapter Two

Blood Testing

Background information

The Diabetes Control and Complications Trial (DCCT) was a 10-year study undertaken from 1983 to 1993 (funded by the American organisation, the National Institute of Diabetes and Digestive and Kidney Diseases) in order to assess the effects of intensive therapy on the long-term complications of diabetes.

The study very clearly showed that intensive management (i.e. close control) of insulin-dependent diabetes prevents or slows the development of the long-term complications of diabetes (possible eye, kidney and nerve damage). Blood tests and frequent insulin doses (for Type 1 diabetics) are part of this close control and are necessary to avoid the onset of diabetic complications.

What is a blood test, how do I do one and why should I bother?

Diabetes is about having higher than normal levels of sugar in the blood, which can usually be controlled with medication. High blood sugars can lead to damage in the body.

A diagnosis of diabetes will be made based on several blood test results showing abnormally high results. After diagnosis you may need to do blood tests on a day-to-day basis so you know what is happening in your body.

For a blood test you will need:

- A blood test machine.

- A blood test strip (or sensor).
- A lancing device.

It is also good practice to have a blood glucose diary to hand so you can record your results. (See page 123 for an example.)

Blood test machines (or blood glucose meters)

Today there is a wide choice of personal blood test machines available and one will easily suit your needs (see chapter 8 on diabetes equipment). They are easy to use and you'll soon get the hang of using one. Your diabetes nurse should be able to offer you advice and may give you a free blood test machine when you are diagnosed. They come with instructions and many have a helpline phone number to call if you are having difficulties.

Modern blood test machines are an invaluable tool for helping you to control your condition. Most now have memories, so if you're not able to write down your blood test results, you can write them down later or even download them onto a PC (see 'choosing a blood test machine' in chapter 8).

If you have Type 1 diabetes you'd be well advised to get a spare blood test machine if you can. It's good to have one somewhere handy during the day e.g. in your bag, desk drawer or glove compartment, as well as one at home. It's also good to know you have one spare in case something happens to your original meter. You can buy them in a pharmacy for less than £20, which is a small investment for your peace of mind and your overall health.

'Today there is a wide choice of personal blood test machines available and one will easily suit your needs. They are easy to use and you'll soon get the hang of using one.'

Blood test sensors

Blood test sensors (also called blood test strips or electrodes) are available on prescription from your GP and are free. You may need to get a Medical Exemption Certificate in order to get your prescriptions for free (see glossary) and you may need to discuss how many sensors you are likely to need based on your suggested blood testing regime. If you're doing five-a-day, then you'll be using 35 sensors a week. Most come in little pots of around 20 sensors, so you may need more than one pot a week.

In addition, your doctor is likely to do a HbA1c test as well (see page 24 for further information).

Lancets

No one likes blood tests, but they are not that bad. Lancets are blood sampling devices that prick the skin to obtain a sample. Things have certainly improved over the years; lancets are sharper, therefore quite painless, and offer a choice of grades that adjust the depth to which they pierce the skin – so whether you're blood testing a child or you're a builder with thick skin on your fingers, there will be a depth that suits you.

In the main, you will probably use the lancing device that comes with your blood test machine. However, many people stick with their old lancing device when they get a new machine, or stick with the machine that has the best lancing device for them.

Blood testing sites

The main sites used for drawing a drop of blood for use in a blood test are the ends of your fingers, which are also well-known for being very sensitive! Try to use the edges of your fingertips (not the top of your fingertips) as these tend to be a little less sensitive.

Some machines are okay if you use Alternative Testing Sites (ATS). This may be the forearm or other areas where blood can be easily obtained. For small children, the earlobe might be used.

Whatever site you prefer, try not to keep using the same one over and over again. As with insulin injection sites, you are better off if you rotate your sites – you'll soon make a site very sore if you keep using it, so make it a habit to use different places on your fingers and alternate the finger you use for blood testing.

'As with insulin injection sites, you are better off if you rotate your sites – you'll soon make a site very sore if you keep using it, so make it a habit to use different places on your fingers and alternate the finger you use for blood testing.'

Blood test frequency

For people with Type 1 diabetes (also known as insulin dependent diabetes) it's recommended that you test your blood sugar at least three times a day, normally before each meal. Any change in routine – exercising more than normal, eating less than usual, travelling or if you are ill – is another good reason to test your blood sugar.

If you have Type 2, which means you take oral medication alone or oral medication as well as insulin to manage your diabetes, you may only need to test your blood sugar once a day. If you're able to control your blood sugar without medication and just with diet and exercise, you may only need to test your blood sugar once a week.

Blood test results

For non-diabetics, normal blood sugar levels are approximately between 4.0 and 8.0 millimoles per litre (mmols/L). If you have diabetes you may not get 'normal' results that often. If you are under 4.0 mmols/L then you are hypoglycaemic and have a low blood sugar. If you are over 8.0 mmols/L then you are hyperglycaemic and have high blood sugar.

Gaining good blood glucose control is the best way to avoid any of the extremely unpleasant complications associated with diabetes (damage to kidneys, eyes and feet). Do as many blood tests as recommended by your diabetes team and try to get used to writing them down so that you can assess them. But please do not get discouraged or frightened by bad results – we all get them.

One of the downsides of multiple blood tests is the amount of information you get – it can result in information overload and you can't see the wood for the trees. So many results, but what does it all mean? You need to be able to see your results with an analytical eye – if the results are not within the normal range, then why was it high, why was it low? It's only by beginning to understand your results that you can start to improve them.

Also, it's possible to overdo it – you should regularly do three or four tests a day, not a test every 30 minutes. For good control, you need to be looking at patterns – are you always high after breakfast? If so, you may need to take more insulin with your breakfast. Writing down your results, especially in a good diary that lets you see how your blood sugar varies throughout the day, can be very helpful.

Interpreting your results

This is best done by writing them down. But it's not just the blood test results, it's the results plus your medication and doses, as well as what you have been eating, what time of day or night it is and what your activity levels have been.

You can discuss this with your diabetes team, but gaining your own understanding is desirable. It's a tall order, but don't be dismayed. It is vital for you to really understand what's happening with your blood sugars, especially if you're newly diagnosed with Type 1 diabetes or having a rough time of it.

If some of your readings are too high or too low, you should consider some or all of the following when trying to understand your results:

1. Time. Your blood test results are likely to be higher in the first hour or so after you have eaten. They are likely to be lower before mealtimes.

2. Food. Your results will reflect when you last ate and the nature of what you ate (in terms of the Glycaemic Index of the food you have eaten – see page 54).

3. Medication. If you get a series of high or low blood sugars (e.g. you are always high before lunchtime) it may reflect that you need more medication (in this case, with your breakfast).

I was told a story about a woman who used to get hypos regularly every Friday during the late morning. It turned out that she was having an insulin injection in her arm in the morning and then cleaning her windows. The extra exercise would make the insulin absorb faster. She was advised to take less insulin on days she was about to attempt lengthy domestic chores. Getting to know your own individual needs like this will develop over time.

The HbA1c blood test

The HbA1c is a blood test that your doctor or nurse will do. Many diabetics see this as the Holy Grail – it's the number that you need to focus on as it is a very good indication of the likelihood of developing diabetic complications. The results may take a week or two to come through, unless your GP or hospital has the appropriate blood test machine for this purpose. The result is in the same range as your normal blood test result, but it's different in that it shows your blood glucose average for up to the last three months.

HbA1c is a measure of glycosylated (or glycated) haemoglobin (it's often called haemoglobin A1c, Hb1c or HbA1c). Glycation of haemoglobin has been implicated in kidney disease and eye damage in diabetes.

Monitoring the HbA1c (also known as Average BG) in diabetics may improve treatment. Higher levels of HbA1c are found in people with persistently elevated blood sugar. A diabetic with good glucose control has a HbA1c level that is close to or within the reference range of between 4%–6.5%. High blood sugars – and therefore high HbA1c results – increase the risk for the long-term complications of diabetes.

The HbA1c is only an average; you should also be looking at avoiding having your blood sugars rocketing from very low to very high, or vice-versa. The more steady and stable your blood sugars are, the less damage there is being caused.

'The HbA1c is a blood test that your doctor or nurse will do. Many diabetics see this as the Holy Grail – it's the number that you need to focus on as it is a very good indication of the likelihood of developing diabetic complications.'

Summing Up

- Talk to your practice nurse or your diabetes nurse about which blood test machine they recommend for you and how often you should test.

- Keeping a blood test diary can be very useful, especially for the newly diagnosed or anyone going through a rough patch with their diabetes control.

- Your diabetes does not care if you are busy – you need to make time to look after yourself, so start to schedule blood tests into your day. Testing before eating is a good guideline for all Type 1s, and Type 2s on insulin.

- Don't be frightened of 'bad' results. We all get them. Just learn to interpret why you've had a high (or a low) and learn how to avoid them.

Chapter Three

Medications Explained

Diet and pill therapy

If you are diagnosed with any form of diabetes, you are going to have to take a long hard look at your diet and eating habits. Your diet is just what you eat and drink – 'being on a diet' is different. As it's a genetic condition, Type 1 diabetes can affect even the healthiest people who have great diets.

However, most Type 2 diabetes (about 80%) is related to being overweight, so if you are diagnosed with Type 2 diabetes you may initially be started on diet therapy, often with some pills added to help control various symptoms. If this is not successful, insulin therapy may also be introduced. Success is judged on blood test results.

Diabetes management

The key point to remember is that diabetes management is a marathon not a sprint.

People with Type 2 diabetes tend to have two problems: they don't make quite enough insulin, and the cells of their bodies don't seem to take in glucose as eagerly as they should. The drugs detailed overleaf manage Type 2 diabetes in different ways to help diabetics maintain good blood glucose control.

Sometimes it's recommended that you take more than one of these different drugs, and it's possible that after a few years their effectiveness may reduce and you may need to review which drugs you are taking. Remember, the information in this book is only a broad guide - you are strongly advised to talk to your GP for professional medical advice and information.

'The key point to remember is that diabetes management is a marathon not a sprint.'

Sulfonylureas

These medications are the oldest of the tablets available. Tolinase (tolazamide) has been around since the 1950s and is still prescribed. Newer drugs in this class include Glucotrol (glipizide), Glucotrol XL (glipizide extended release), Amaryl (glimepiride), Diabeta (glyburide) and Micronase (glyburide). These allow the pancreas to release more insulin, which lowers the glucose level, but hypoglycemia is a common side effect. Many of these drugs are only effective for a few years.

Biguanides

These drugs work by affecting the production of glucose that comes from digestion. They lower cholesterol numbers, help with weight loss and don't cause hypoglycemia. They are the most commonly prescribed drugs for Type 2 diabetes. Glucophage (metformin) and Glucophage XR (metformin extended release) are the most well known of these drugs.

Metformin lowers blood glucose levels primarily by decreasing the amount of glucose produced by the liver. Metformin also helps to lower blood glucose levels by making muscle tissue more sensitive to insulin so glucose can be absorbed. It is usually taken two times a day. A side effect of metformin may be diarrhoea, but this is improved when the drug is taken with food.

Alpha-Glucosidase Inhibitors

Glyset (miglitol) and Precose (acarbose) are the two most prescribed alpha-glucosidase inhibitors (also known as 'starch blockers'). These drugs help the body to lower blood glucose levels by blocking the breakdown of starches (such as bread, potatoes and pasta) in the intestine. They also slow the breakdown of some sugars such as basic granulated sugar.

These medications need to be taken at the beginning of each meal so that they can work to slow digestion, which in turn slows the rise of glucose in the blood. They are often prescribed in conjunction with other diabetes medications and they may cause diarrhoea or gas.

Thiazolidinediones

These drugs work by sensitising muscle and fat cells to accept insulin more readily. Actos (pioglitazone) and Avandia (rosiglitazone) are the only two thiazolidinediones marketed today. However, in 2007, the Food and Drug Administration (FDA) in the USA issued a safety alert regarding the possibility of heart attacks or other fatal cardiovascular events when taking Avandia.

Meglitinides

Also taken before each meal, these drugs stimulate the pancreas to produce more insulin in relationship to how much glucose is in the blood. The brand names for these drugs are Prandin (repaglinide) and Starlix (nateglinide). They can be used in combination with some other oral medications for increased effectiveness.

DPP-4 Inhibitors

A new oral medication called Januvia (sitagliptin phosphate) has been approved in the USA for management of Type 2 diabetes. It's the first in a new class of drugs called DPP-4 Inhibitors. Januvia lowers blood sugar levels by blocking an enzyme known as Dipeptidyl Peptidase IV or DPP-4. Januvia showed good results in recent trials – both in combination with other drugs like metformin and also by itself.

Insulin

For Type 1 diabetics insulin injections are an unavoidable means to control the condition. However, Type 2 diabetics are increasingly being put on insulin therapy as a means of treating diabetes. Going onto insulin takes some getting used to but you're only doing it to gain better control, so there's little point in resenting it. It is not a failure to end up on insulin, nor is it a sign that your diabetes is getting worse. It's just that insulin therapy is the best treatment for your condition at that time.

The medical equipment that goes with insulin therapy (blood test machines, lancing devices, needles and insulin pens) are all of great quality these days. In particular, lancing devices and needles are smaller, sharper and less painful than they used to be, so count yourself lucky!

In the USA, insulin is advertised on the TV – it would be your decision to discuss using it as part of your diabetes treatment. In the UK, there's no such link between the manufacturer and the patient, so it's good to ask questions to find out about how insulin may help you.

The proof that it is helping (and is worth it) will be your blood test results.

Insulin therapy

There are various brands and forms of insulin available and your diabetes team will guide you through what you need to use. This may take quite a bit of time to get right once you are first diagnosed, so be patient and vigilant – make sure you ask questions about your medication and dosage. Essentially it can take a while for you and your medication to 'settle down'. Over the years, your medicine usage may change due to your age, your time of life and other factors.

The main forms of insulin available are:

- Rapid-acting insulin begins working within 15 minutes and its action lasts a few hours.

- Short-acting insulin takes 30 to 45 minutes to work and lasts a few hours.

- Intermediate-acting insulin is mixed with a substance that causes the body to absorb the insulin more slowly. It begins to work within two to four hours.

- Long-acting (basal) insulin acts in a way that is more or less stable for the whole day. It's often referred to as 24-hour insulin as its release and effectiveness often lasts a whole day.

Most adults on insulin take a long-acting and a short-acting insulin. There is a simple logic to this – it's the best way to imitate what a non-diabetic's body does.

Non-diabetics have a certain amount of insulin present at all times, but when they eat, a larger amount of insulin is used as part of a feedback mechanism within the body. The pituitary gland in the brain constantly measures blood sugar levels. If the levels are too low, glucagon is released in order to raise blood sugar levels. If the levels are too high, insulin is released in order to lower those levels.

If you are on insulin then you will have to start doing the work of your pituitary gland by doing a blood test to see what your blood glucose level is. Then you figure out how much insulin you need and give yourself a dose.

Short-acting and long-acting insulin

Different insulins have been made to help people with diabetes. Each works slightly differently with its own release pattern. Insulins that get to work fast, do their job and then become inactive within a few hours are called short-acting insulin. This includes such insulins as Humalog from Eli Lilly and Novo Rapid from Novo Nordisk.

Characteristically, these start working within about 10 or 20 minutes of being injected and will have started to wear off after about two hours. The idea is that this mimics the kind of release pattern that occurs in a non-diabetic around meal times. You'll have an injection of short-acting insulin with a meal.

The body needs insulin at all times, it just needs more at meal times. Along with short-acting insulins for mealtimes, you are likely to have a long-acting insulin as well. These include Lantus from Sanofi Aventis and Levemir from Novo Nordisk. By having a long-acting insulin (also known as 24-hour insulin or 'peakless' insulin), you have some insulin present all day long. These long-acting insulins are often the ones given to Type 2 diabetics when their condition requires it.

Going on insulin does not mean your diabetes is worse, though it may mean that the drugs you have been using are no longer working. Insulin therapy will only be suggested if it seems to be the best route to achieve better blood sugar control and therefore avert any possible diabetes complications.

Human or animal insulin

Much insulin today is made by pharmaceutical companies and is called human insulin. Historically, all insulin was animal insulin – literally extracted from the pancreases of either pigs or cows. These porcine or bovine insulins are still available, though they are rarely given out. Some users who moved from animal to human insulin reported serious side effects, most likely attributable to bad calculations of how to convert the dose of animal insulin across to the 'human' version. As you need less human insulin (relatively), wrong conversions could give huge and horrid hypos (which would put any one off). Today, most people take to human insulin very well.

How to look after insulin

'You have to look after your insulin, so you need to get used to storing it the right way and using it correctly.'

You have to look after your insulin, so you need to get used to storing it the right way and using it correctly. It has a use-by-date on it which must be checked when you go to start a new bottle of insulin or cartridge. See the instructions that come with your insulin or talk to your GP or pharmacist for advice on insulin storage.

Basically, when not in use, insulin should be kept in the refrigerator. Insulin MUST NOT be frozen as this will deactivate it. Also avoid high temperatures as this can impair it. When in use (in your insulin pen or in your bag), try to keep your insulin in a dry place at room temperature and out of sunlight. Once it is opened it is generally recommended that insulin should be used within 28 days, whether it is refrigerated or not.

Damaged insulin

Short-acting insulin that is cloudy, clumped or crystallised may be inactive – seek medical advice and do not take it. Long-acting insulins are normally cloudy, so look for clumping or crystallisation as a sign of it being damaged. Talk to your GP for advice.

Which insulin is best for me?

This will be determined by your diabetes team in discussion with you, but may depend on some or all of the following factors:

- Your other health requirements such as exercise, diet and other medications.
- Your ability to perform glucose monitoring and your level of comfort with multiple injections (though you have no choice if you're Type 1 – you have to inject insulin and you are well advised to do blood tests).
- Your age.
- Which insulin will suit you best based on its action (how soon it starts to work, its peak in terms of action and how long it lasts).
- Your individual response to insulin.

Insulin dosage

This is going to be a very important part of your diabetes management and control of blood sugar levels. If you get it right, your blood test results will be in the recommended range of between 4.0 mmols/L and 8.0 mmols/L (probably a little higher just after eating). Getting this right is very hard, so don't be disheartened if you get readings that are out of the recommended range, but try to keep at it. Good control reduces the chances of complications, and achieving this will be a central part of your daily life.

Your dose will depend on the following:

- Your blood test result.
- How much and what type of food you are about to have.
- If you are about to do exercise.

One of the tools that many people with diabetes use is 'carbohydrate counting'. This gives an idea of the total carbohydrates you are about to have. There are guidelines as to how much insulin to use to cover the carbohydrates – you may do one unit of insulin to every 10g of carbohydrates. See page 53 for more information on counting carbohydrates.

'One of the tools that many people with diabetes use is "carbohydrate counting". This gives an idea of the total carbohydrates you are about to have.'

However, while this sounds simple, there are variables that can affect the dose, including your weight, height and what the food is that you are about to eat. Each diabetic needs different amounts of insulin, so you may find that you have to do four units of insulin for each 10g of carbohydrate. Or, if you are eating a carbohydrate that is combined with fat (think of chips), the fat affects how and when the chips are absorbed. In this case, you may find you need more insulin and that the absorption of the chips takes more than the two hours your insulin works for, so you may need to do an extra injection later on.

Getting used to how you react to different foods will help you understand how you need to adjust your insulin (or what foods to avoid). In the UK, there are diabetes education programmes called DAFNE (for Type 1s) and DESMOND (for Type 2s), both of which feature information on counting carbohydrates. Ask your diabetes team about access to these courses (for more information, see pages 97 and 98).

Tips on how to take insulin

Some doctors suggest taking insulin 20 minutes before having your meal. However, it can be safer to see your food before you assess your dose. After ordering food in a restaurant, I've had an injection only to then find that the food was not what I had expected. Then I've had to ask for extra bread to 'mop up' the excess insulin I'd already injected. Once it's 'in', it's going to do exactly what it is designed to do, so see your food first, before deciding on your dose.

Digestion also does take a little bit of time to get going, so it's likely that the insulin action will have started by the time the energy from your food is coming into your blood stream and the two should balance each other out.

The time you take your insulin – for example 20 minutes before you eat or just a moment before you start to eat – will depend a lot upon the 'action' of insulin – how long it takes to become active in your body and how long that action lasts (covered in more detail on page 31).

Talk to your GP or medical team for advice.

Factfile

- Insulin is not swallowed because stomach acid destroys it, though researchers are trying to create insulin pills that overcome this obstacle.

- Insulin is delivered via needle-and-syringe injections, insulin pens, jet injectors or insulin pumps. A recent attempt for an inhaled insulin resulted in Exubera, which was delivered into the nose by a sort of pump. This did not prove popular as the pump was big and would have drawn too much attention to anyone using it.

- Remember that different locations on the body absorb insulin at different rates. The best site is the tummy because insulin is absorbed most consistently from there.

- It might be a good idea to use your tummy or arms for short-acting insulin doses and your legs for long-acting insulin. Basically, don't inject long-acting insulins in the same site as the short-acting – it could affect the absorption capabilities of both.

- Rotate the injection sites you use – don't keep putting injections into the same spot. If you do this, you'll get sore as you're damaging the area with multiple injections. It also means that the insulin may not absorb at a constant rate.

- Likely sites are: upper arm, outer or inner thighs, top of the buttocks and the stomach.

- When combining insulins in an injection, inject the insulin within five minutes of mixing.

Other drugs

ACE inhibitors

ACE inhibitors, or inhibitors of Angiotensin-Converting Enzyme, are a group of drugs that are used mainly in the treatment of hypertension (high blood pressure) and congestive heart failure. These may be prescribed for you if you have signs of renal disease (protein in your urine) or for the prevention of kidney disease.

Statins

Statins are cholesterol lowering tablets. They are a class of drugs that lower the level of cholesterol in the blood by reducing the production of cholesterol by the liver. This is because statins block the enzyme in the liver that is responsible for making cholesterol.

Statins, like ACE inhibitors, are an important class of drugs because they have been shown to reduce the incidence of heart attacks, strokes and death. Doctors consider giving statins to anyone with diabetes who has a substantial risk of heart attack or stroke.

Summing Up

- Any new medication will take a bit of getting used to. Allow yourself some space to get doses right, no matter what medication you are given.

- Always take your insulin – if you are ill or off your food for any reason, you can reduce it. Just don't go without it – you'll regret it!

- Look after your medications as per the instructions and keep out of the reach of children. For insulin – avoid extremes of heat or cold. If travelling, do not put insulin in luggage that goes in the hold (as it can freeze and can become deactivated).

- Talk to your GP for professional medical advice about medication.

Chapter Four

Treating a Hypo or Hyper

Very high (hyperglycaemia) or very low (hypoglycaemia) blood sugar levels can occur in diabetics and need to be treated immediately. A blood test will establish whether you are having a hypo or a hyper. It's easy to find the language a bit of a challenge, but think 'low' and think 'hypo.' To treat a hypo (under 4.0 mmols/L) you are likely to administer a form of sugar, whereas for hyperglycaemia (over 8.0 mmols/L) you could administer insulin or pills.

Not all blood test results over 8.0 mmols/L need to be addressed. If your result is a bit high you should wait and see if it drops before treating it with extra insulin.

A diabetic with a low blood sugar is often said to be 'having a hypo' or 'going hypo'. Diabetics themselves have a range of ways to describe the feeling of having a hypo – often describing it as 'being a bit wobbly'. It's also a medical fact that people having a hypo can act very oddly – it is often associated with giddiness, vision problems and a sudden irritability.

Hypoglycaemia (hypos)

The first thing to say about hypos is that they are pretty much inevitable for someone with diabetes – perhaps even more so if you are well-controlled.

Being well-controlled means mostly having blood test results in the 4.0 – 8.0 mmols/L range, which can be a small window to aim for, particularly if you have Type 1 and you're using blood tests and injected insulin to achieve it. You will often find yourself close to or under the 4.0 mmols/L lower guideline.

But if you're well-controlled then you should have hypo symptoms and good strategies to handle a hypo in the best possible manner.

'Not all blood test results over 8.0 mmols/L need to be addressed. If your result is a bit high you should wait and see if it drops before treating it with extra insulin.'

Hypos: definition and terminology

Normal blood sugars should be between 4.0 – 8.0 mmols/L. A hypo can be defined as being under 4.0 mmols/L. A mild hypo might be a reading of 3.7mmols/L, while a more severe hypo would be so low that the blood test meter you are using may just say 'low', meaning that you're off the scale when it comes to reading a glucose result.

It's a good habit to 'make 4 the floor' – i.e. make 4.0 mmols/L the lowest reading you get. In fact, many diabetics make 5 the floor – if they get a reading of 5.0, they would have a biscuit to avoid going any lower and risking a hypo.

Any diabetic can tell you what they feel when having a hypo – in the main, you get shaky, irritable, find it hard to concentrate and often have a very strong urge to eat anything that you can lay your hands on (I know I do!). Your hypo, and how to treat it, will be very specific to yourself and your needs – how your hypo was induced, where you are, what you last ate, what your activity levels are (or have been) and what you have to hand when the hypo strikes.

Some people get good hypo symptoms – and by good I mean that it is good that you have symptoms, not that it's good that you're having a hypo! It's my belief that hypos should be avoided like the plague for the obvious reasons that they feel bad and because they tend to lead to at least a few hours of 'up and down' blood test results.

One of the big factors in coping with your diabetes is 'keeping your head above water' – it is not easy having diabetes, and having hypos can seriously undermine your confidence in your ability to live with the condition.

Hypo handling

It's very easy to over do it when it comes to treating a hypo and that's one thing you need to get used to handling. Some hypos are worse than others – in as much as they can come on more suddenly or you get to be very low – with a reading of 3.0 mmols/L or lower.

'Any diabetic can tell you what they feel when having a hypo – in the main, you get shaky, irritable, find it hard to concentrate and often have a very strong urge to eat anything that you can lay your hands on. Your hypo, and how to treat it, will be very specific to yourself and your needs.'

You may get to the point when you know your blood sugar level and you know exactly what you need to do to correct it. For example, if you're at 3.5 mmols/L you need a 200ml glass of orange juice or if you're at 2.5 mmols/L you need a glass of orange juice and a mini-Mars bar or two.

The thing that non-diabetics can fail to understand is that you are deeply addled when having a hypo. You are confused, annoyed and perhaps not able to make good decisions or explain yourself well. Let those around you know how a hypo tends to affect you. You're best off keeping them informed so they can be a help not a hindrance. It's very likely that they will be able to tell you are going into one, possibly even before you do.

Advice for parents and guardians

You are really up against it when dealing with young children and hypos. It's hard enough with them having all the various 'phases' of discovering their personality and place in the universe, but you have to keep an eye out and decide when a temper tantrum is in fact a hypo.

Signs you can watch for:

- Sudden snaps of temper might be part and parcel of any child's day (they're still part of mine!), but signs to watch for are if they are looking pale (or 'peaky') and are being more irrational than normal.

- Another tip is to ask them to hold their hand out and see if it shakes when they do so.

- If a few of these signs are present you can assume your child is going hypo. Try to do a blood test to confirm it, but otherwise treat it as a hypo.

Teachers and work colleagues should be aware of what a hypo is and how to help the person having one. That might mean knowing how it happens and where the diabetic keeps their blood test machine (and even knowing how to use it), as well as having some sugar to hand.

'Teachers and work colleagues should be aware of what a hypo is and how to help the person having one. That might mean knowing how it happens and where the diabetic keeps their blood test machine (and even knowing how to use it), as well as having some sugar to hand.'

Hypo treatments

The lower the reading, the more sugar you will need to 'pull yourself out of it'. Treatment is also known simply as a 'sugar source' because any sugar can be a hypo treatment, but some might be better (faster or more effective) than others.

Nothing can legitimately be claimed to be a hypo treatment until it has been clinically tested, which is true of very few products indeed. Neither sugar, cola, orange juice or chocolate have had clinical trials but, as any diabetic can tell you, they work when it comes to pulling you out of a hypo.

A liquid will work faster in your system than a solid – so smoothies, fruit juice or one of the gluco gel products (see glossary) are a good bet for an initial reaction to a hypo. Solids need a bit of digestion before the sugars are released – they will work, but they'll just take a bit longer to do so.

Likewise, a boiled sweet will take longer to deliver than say a chewy toffee or a crunchable tablet.

A list of sugar sources

I'm listing these as a sort of scale, with the most dramatic hypo-stoppers at the top and the weaker ones at the bottom. The amount of response required to treat the hypo will be indicated by the severity of the hypo (so do a blood test to find out what you're dealing with).

Glucagon injection (GlucaGen HypoKit): this is for someone in a bad hypo, possibly past the point of being able to help themselves (who may be unconscious). It's an injection that contains glucagon – a pure form of energy that gets straight into the system without having to be digested. You can get these on prescription from your GP. Keep refrigerated when not in use and do not use when any other hypo treatments are available.

Fruit juices and smoothies: astonishingly sugary (as sugary as a cola – read the labels!), but there's a sense that they're healthier than a fizzy drink.

Soft drinks: good, but fizzy ones can be quite harsh on the throat if you need to drink them quickly.

Sugar cubes: old-fashioned but easy; keep a box handy for emergencies.

Gluco-tabs: available from Boots and larger pharmacies, these are glucose tablets that you can chew to release energy, with 4g of glucose in each tablet. They now come in a handy little plastic tube carrying 10 'tabs' which can be refilled from a bigger bottle. The small tube is around 80p, the bigger bottle under £3.00. New on the market is Gluco Juice - little bottles of 15g of carbohydrate in liquid form.

Hypo-fit: a syrup packed in foil sachets, each containing 13g of useful carbohydrate. As syrup, these are even easier than chewing a tab. The foil sachets are durable, light to carry and do not 'go off'.

Top tips on handling a hypo

1. Make sure you have sugar sources stashed everywhere (a drawer next to your bed, in the glove-compartment of the car, in a desk drawer at work, in your briefcase, handbag or rucksack). Make sure no one feels they can help themselves to these – they are yours for emergencies.

2. Tell those close to you what the symptoms are and how they can help you if you're having a hypo. You should tell at least one colleague how you handle your hypos, just in case you have a diabetes-induced wobbler at work.

3. Try to do a blood test if you can. I know that for me, feeling very anxious can feel very much like a hypo (there is a certain amount of interaction between adrenalin and insulin), but adding sugar to anxiety won't help at all while adding sugar to a hypo will. So know what you're dealing with.

4. Try to treat the hypo with something very sugary (sweets, orange juice, cola or other soft drinks), as well as something more long-term (a biscuit or a slice of bread which will release its sugars over a longer period of time). But don't overdo it.

5. Read the label on whatever you're using to treat the hypo so you know how much energy you are putting in.

6. Wait 10 minutes and do another blood test and see if you need more anti-hypo action.

7. Test again about an hour later. By then, if you've overdone it, you might need a little insulin 'chaser' to bring down a high sugar, but be careful – you don't want to end up having another hypo!

8. Try to keep note of when you have hypos – if there is a pattern (for example, you get lows at 10.30am every weekday) then it may indicate that you need to adjust your medication or change what or when you are eating.

9. Have a back-up blood test machine to keep in your bedroom in case you can't sleep and are worrying it might be because your sugars are low, or if you actually wake up feeling hypo. Keep some sugar near you to deal with the hypo as soon as you can – going to another room, especially up or downstairs when you're 'wobbly', can be more of a challenge than normal. Ask for one at your clinic or buy one – you can get them for less than £20 at a pharmacy.

Remember to replace the sugar sources that you use up. Preparation is all! It's bad enough having a hypo without having a panic attack too.

'Remember to replace the sugar sources that you use up. Preparation is all! It's bad enough having a hypo without having a panic attack too.'

Post-hypo analysis

See if you can rationalise why the hypo happened.

- Did you take too much insulin or eat too few carbohydrates?
- Did you take unexpected exercise after your meal?
- Can you avoid repeating the same circumstances and having another hypo?

See the diary at the end of this book for more help with this.

Hyperglycaemia and ketoacidosis

Hyperglycaemia is right at the other end of the scale and is when you have a high blood sugar. This tends to feel less dramatic (unless it's untreated, in which case it can end up with hospitalisation). Many diabetics find unexpected or unexplained high blood sugars very distressing, especially if they're trying hard to achieve good control.

Remember though – not all blood test results over 8.0 mmols/L need to be addressed. If your result is 9.0 or 10 mmols/L you should wait and see if it drops before treating it with extra insulin.

The likely symptoms of hyperglycaemia will be: feeling thirsty, feeling tired, generally not feeling well and having to go to the toilet a lot to urinate. Depending on the medication, this can be addressed by taking a small shot of insulin. If unaddressed, this might result in what is often called a sugar coma (or diabetic coma), which is a result of ketoacidosis (see below). If left untreated, you can lose consciousness and will need hospitalisation to regain control and consciousness.

Ketoacidosis is a process that begins in the body when the blood sugars are very high. It involves the breaking down of body fat in order to release energy for the body to use. This is the body going into an emergency back-up situation – it's not designed to sustain this for long and essentially it becomes toxic to the body.

The by-product of this breakdown are ketones, which can build up and start to affect brain function. It's ironic that the diabetic is suffering from the impact high sugars have and yet the body cannot access these sugars as it needs insulin in order to do so. The patient will become dehydrated and can literally just waste away unless there is medical intervention (this is what people with diabetes used to die of before insulin was discovered by Banting and Bets in 1919).

There are guidelines which say that if a diabetic does a blood test and it's higher than 12.0 mmols/L, they should also test for ketones. Some test machines are available that test for ketones – one even tests blood and ketones (with separate strips).

The fact is, if you have relatively well-controlled diabetes you should not need to worry about ketones. However, if you do start getting ketone readings you may want to talk it over with your diabetes team. The only way to treat the ketoacidosis is to get back to good diabetes control with sugars under 10 mmols/L but over 4.0 mmols/L.

Please be aware that if you are ill your body is likely to have slightly raised blood sugars as a result. However, don't stop taking your medication. You may need to cut it back, especially if you are off your food, but do not stop taking it! (See page 106).

'Please be aware that if you are ill your body is likely to have slightly raised blood sugars as a result. However, don't stop taking your medication. You may need to cut it back, especially if you are off your food, but do not stop taking it!'

Summing Up

- Hypos (low blood sugars) are somewhat inevitable, especially with insulin therapy. Trying to have 'tight' control means being close to the line (the lower blood test reading you can have before you are considered to be in a hypo is 4.0 mmols/L).

- Be prepared – keep a sugar source or hypo treatment at home, in the office, at school and in the car, ideally along with a blood test machine.

- Try not to 'blow your socks off' when treating a hypo. Hypos make you feel like you should eat everything you can lay your hands on, but that will result in a very high blood sugar which is no good either. Gently does it – steady as she goes!

- Tell those close to you what it feels like to have a hypo and how a hypo affects you – they might need to help you if you get confused or angry (both of which are symptoms of hypos).

- Do a blood test if you feel like you have low blood sugar – it might just be a feeling of being stressed (with similar feelings of anxiety and shaking).

- If you have a series of very high blood test readings, seek medical advice – hyperglycaemia (high blood sugar) can also be dangerous.

Chapter Five

Diabetes and Diet

Is there a diabetic diet?

There seems to be a lot of people who don't like to think there is such a thing as 'the diabetic diet'. There is no set diet – that much is clear – but it's more like a series of guidelines for eating. The great thing about these recommendations is that they are about as healthy as it gets – low in sugar, low in fat, and with plenty of variation allowed within these parameters.

When you are first diagnosed with diabetes you will have help from a specialist dietician who will give you information on which foods are better for you. But you also need to educate yourself about food and learn about your own body's reactions to food stuff. We each react a little differently to foods, so you will have to assess how you are getting on by doing a blood test.

The food pyramid

The food pyramid is used more in the USA than in the UK, but the idea is to show a recommended intake across the food groups. You can see from the diagram overleaf that you should eat a variety of foods. It also shows that you should eat less of some foods (those at the top of the pyramid) and more of others (the ones at the bottom).

A balanced diet is one that includes all the food groups. In other words, you should have foods from every colour, every day. Each colour of vegetable and fruit has different benefits, and eating a broad range of colours ensures you are getting all the nutrients you need. You might have heard of 'eat a rainbow', which is the same idea.

'You need to educate yourself about food and learn about your own body's reactions to food stuff. We each react a little differently to foods, so you will have to assess how you are getting on by doing a blood test.'

The food pyramid

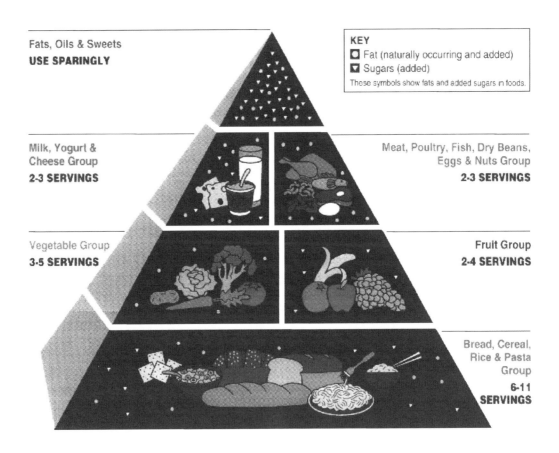

Source: Wikimedia Commons

However, eating from all of the food categories does not guarantee weight loss. If you are interested in losing weight, you need to be concerned with calorie intake while eating foods in each food group. Try choosing low-fat or non-fat varieties of food when available and cook with little oil and butter. Also, try not to think that you should eat a lot of bread, pasta, rice and cereals just because they're in the 'biggest' slice of the pyramid. Have some with each meal, but too many carbohydrates will lead to weight gain.

Finally, don't forget that the food pyramid is only a guideline!

Blood testing

- Type 2 diabetes – you may only need to test once a day or once a week as Type 2 is often considered to be easier to control. That doesn't mean to say that you won't have a lot to get to grips with in your diet.

- Type 1 diabetes – you are likely to be encouraged to blood test before each meal and before bedtime, and at each of these points in time you are likely to have both an injection and something to eat.

Highs and lows

When you have diabetes you will see how food affects you with much greater clarity than someone without diabetes. If your medication and your food don't balance each other out, your blood sugar level will either be too high or too low. Both can make you feel under par and can, in extreme instances, be dangerous.

Getting your diabetic control right can be a time-consuming and arduous task, especially as it concerns absolutely everything you eat, drink and do. Keep doing blood tests though – this is the only way you'll know if you're achieving good control.

For the newly diagnosed, it's particularly difficult – you are new to it all and therefore unfamiliar with it. You will also be wrestling with new medications and finding the right doses, which might take some time to sort out.

Remember though, even those of us who've had the condition for a long time can go through patches where our control isn't good and we have to go back to basics to get it stable again. We all get some unexpected highs or lows that we have to deal with, so don't beat yourself up if you're finding it hard.

Counting carbohydrates & DAFNE

DAFNE (Dose Adjustment For Normal Eating) is a course that incorporates teaching carbohydrate counting for people with Type 1 diabetes. See page 97 for more information.

Carbohydrate counting is a tool that many diabetics use to try and gauge how many carbohydrates they are about to eat as it helps with working out how much insulin is needed. It is not a direct match necessarily, but it's a very good guide.

You will work out with your doctor what your initial medications and doses will be, but it may take some trial and error to get the balance right for you.

The body cannot process carbohydrates unless insulin is present, so it's likely that if you are having a snack of more than 20g of carbohydrates you may (if you're on insuliln) need to take a small shot of insulin as well so that your body can process the carbohydrates. It's a constant balancing act.

'The type of food you eat and the amount of food you eat determine how high and how fast your blood sugar level goes up. Carbohydrate in food affects your blood glucose the most.'

Carboyhdrate value of different foods

Food		Carbohydrates
Baked beans	3 tablespoons (120g)	20
Red kidney beans	3 tablespoons (105g)	20
Butter beans	3 tablespoons (105g)	20
Chick peas cooked	2-3 tablespoons (90g)	15
Red split lentils cooked	2 tablespoons (80g)	15
Dahl, cooked	2 tablespoons	15
Potatoes, boiled	1 average (60g)	10
New potatoes with skin, boiled	1 average (40g)	5
Baked potato with skin	1 medium (180g)	55
Chips	Per 5 chips (50g)	10
Roast potato	1 small (50g)	10
Mashed potatoes	1 scoop (60g) 2 tablespoons (90g)	10 15

From Leeds Teaching Hospitals NHS Trust website www.leedsth.nhs.uk/sites/diabetes.

What are carbohydrates?

Carbohydrates are chains of sugar molecules that are hooked together. Smaller chains are known as simple carbohydrates while longer chains are called complex carbohydrates. Simple carbohydrates naturally occur in fruits, vegetables and milk products, as well as in processed sugars such as sweets, honey, sugar and syrups. Complex carbohydrates are starches found in breads, cereals, rice and pastas. Carbohydrate is broken down into glucose during digestion and this raises blood sugar levels.

Carbohydrate counting explained

The following is taken from the Leeds Teaching Hospitals NHS Trust website (www.leedsteachinghospitals.com), which explains carbohydrate counting very well and has excellent resources for diabetics, including carbohydrate reference tables for food.

- 'Carbohydrate counting means estimating the amount of carbohydrate you are eating. It can be used by everybody, whether on flexible insulin regimes or more fixed doses.

- Counting carbohydrate can help you to adjust your insulin doses or help explain erratic blood sugars.

- The amount of insulin you need per 10g of carbohydrate will vary between individuals – ask your dietician, nurse or clinician.

- More information is available from food labels. Remember, this should be the total carbohydrate content including both starches and sugars.

- It is not an exact science! Rounding up or down to the nearest 5g is acceptable.

To help you work out when and where changes are needed, you will sometimes need to keep records of the foods you eat, your blood glucose and your units of insulin. Knowing about the carbohydrate content of the food and drinks you consume will help you to calculate the amount of insulin you need to achieve better blood glucose levels. Important goals for meal planning are about the right amount of calories based on age/sex/level of activity, and healthy food choices.'

For further information, see www.leedsteachinghospitals.com/sites/diabetes/food/.

There are also guidelines for matching carbohydrate amounts with insulin doses, although these vary widely among diabetics. It does not mean anything specific if you take a certain amount of insulin – people's needs vary from one individual to another.

As an example, some people can simply have one unit of insulin for each 10g of carbohydrate (sometimes 10g of carbohydrate is referred to as one carbohydrate exchange). One unit of insulin per 10g of carbohydrate is a 1:1 ratio of insulin: carbohydrate. So, if your meal is just a sandwich, it's likely to be 50g of carbohydrate, so the insulin dose would be five units. For someone whose ratio is 2:1 (two units of insulin for each 10g of carbohydrate), you would take 10 units of insulin for the same 50g of carbohydrate.

Of course, it's not that simple for everyone. Most people will learn that they may start the day with a 1:1 ratio, but by lunchtime this will have moved to 2:1 and will be at 1 ½:1 for dinner.

This is pretty high-end or 'hardcore' diabetes theory – it's taught in the DAFNE courses and is not widely known about. See the food and blood test diary on page 123 for more help with this.

You might learn that certain foods get digested quite quickly and can make your blood sugars rise fast. Likewise, you will learn about which foods seem to give you a slow, steady energy release, which fits nicely with your insulin or pill release pattern. See more about insulin action on page 30.

The Glycaemic Index (GI)

Knowledge is definitely power when it comes to diabetes and diet. The GI diet, which has had a lot of coverage recently, was originally conceived to help people with diabetes understand how the food they eat affects their blood sugar levels.

The GI is a measure of how quickly sugars in foods are released into the blood stream. The index alone is not a diet, but knowing which foods give which peaks can be a great help in maintaining more consistent blood sugar levels.

The GI ranks foods on a scale of one to 100, according to the extent to which foods raise blood glucose levels after ingestion. Carbohydrates that break down quickly during digestion have the highest GI values and are said to be 'fast-acting'. Carbohydrates which break down slowly, releasing glucose gradually into the bloodstream, have low GI factors. These are known as good carbohydrates and form the basis of a low GI diet. A high GI level is 70 and over, a low GI is under 56.

The GI of a food is influenced by a variety of factors including the degree to which a food is processed; how long the food is cooked; the kind of starch, sugar or fibre the food contains and the food's acidity. In general, anything that speeds the rate at which a food is digested and absorbed will raise its GI.

If you want to lose weight, you may find success if you eat a low GI diet because low GI foods ought to delay feelings of hunger. Complex carbohydrates like porridge and bananas have a slow release pattern (or low GI) which gives a more stable blood sugar level over a period of time.

Factfile

The GI has been the subject of scientific research for over 20 years. It was originally developed as a dietary strategy to help people with diabetes gain better control over their blood sugar levels. Dr. David Jenkins, a professor of nutrition at the University of Toronto, Canada, first developed the concept of the GI. His study, 'Glycaemic index of foods: a physiological basis for carbohydrate exchange,' appeared in March 1981. Subsequently, hundreds of clinical studies in the United Kingdom, France, Italy, Canada and Australia have proved the value of the GI. Today the GI is an accepted part of medical nutrition therapy in Canada, Australia and much of Europe. Its use has expanded to include roles in treating obesity, cardiovascular disease and various other health problems.

Glycaemic Load (GL)

The GI only lists individual foods. It lists cheese, it lists tomato and it lists bread. But we all know that these combine to make a cheese and tomato sandwich, which contains protein, fat and carbohydrates.

Most of us eat food in combinations (hamburger and chips, bangers and mash), which leads to an overall Glycaemic Load (cheese plus tomato plus bread = GL).

You might be combining low GI foods (brown bread for example) with higher GI foods (jam) with fat (butter), giving an overall energy release that's a combination of all the elements making up your snack or meal.

Adding fat to a carbohydrate (think chips as opposed to baked potato) slows down (or rather it extends) the time taken by the body to absorb the food. That's why chips are listed as having a different GI to baked potato. It's also why how you cook your food is part of the overall idea of healthy eating.

It sounds confusing, but a diabetic watching their blood sugars, particularly if they are injecting insulin, is able to see what effect certain foods are having on them. If I have a meal that's unusually big or I indulge in a pudding (where I normally abstain or make do with a spoonful of someone else's if they let me), I make the best judgement I can about the food I'm having but will do an extra blood test shortly afterwards to see how I'm doing. Giving myself too much or too little insulin can have undesirable consequences and I would rather be safe than sorry.

Food labels

Labels on foods are a helpful tool for giving you more idea about what you're eating. In the UK, new food labelling guidelines have brought food contents to the fore. The Food Standards Agency (FSA) has been working with food manufacturers to agree a standard set of guidelines for food labelling. It's been a long and often uphill struggle, but it's starting to show some real headway now.

However, be aware that there are many variations in how a company labels its food, for example some only want to list sugars as opposed to carbohydrates. You will need to know the carbohydrate count, so don't just look at the sugar listing. Also, some labels only give amounts on a per 100g of product basis, which means some challenging mathematics if you have a 27g cereal bar! Be careful and check labels – they can be very useful in helping to handle diabetes.

Guideline Daily Amounts (GDAs)

Each day	Women	Men
Calories	2,000	2,500
Fat	70g	95g
Of which saturates	20g	30g
Protein	45g	55g
Sodium	2.4g	2.4g
Equivalent as salt	6g	6g
Carbohydrate	230g	300g
Sugars	90g	120g

Source: Institute of Grocery Distribution, www.igd.com.

This table shows typical guidelines for Guideline Daily Amounts. Many more food manufacturers are now including helpful labels on their foods. The most useful of these show how much of the GDA of, say, fat is contained in that food. If it was a cereal bar, the label might say that the bar represents 5% of your GDA of fat. Watch out for foods (or food brands or even supermarkets) that do have useful labels; they really can help to reduce the amount of figuring out you have to do about what you eat. I would rather buy a brand with good labelling on it than one without. I vote with my purse!

The traffic light system

In this system, the traffic light colours (red, amber and green) are used to help you get the balance right by helping you to choose between products and keep a check on the high-fat, high-sugar and high-salt foods you eat. Green is for foods that are low GI, orange (or amber) is for moderate release sugars and red is for foods with a relatively high sugar content.

The traffic light colours can make it easier for you to compare products at a glance. If the label tells you how much of the nutrient is in a portion, this can also help you to compare products. You might be surprised how much difference there can be between similar products. However, if your favourite foods get some red traffic lights, it's still fine to have them occasionally!

Visit the FSAs site at www.eatwell.gov.uk/foodlabels/trafficlights for more information. Few manufacturers have joined this scheme and in the UK it is voluntary.

The What's Inside Guide

This guide is another new labelling system being introduced across foods and drinks in the UK.

These at-a-glance labels tell you how many calories, sugars, fat, saturates and salt there are in what you're about to eat, including a reference to your Guideline Daily Amounts (GDAs). The labels can be used to take the guesswork out of what we should be eating and make planning a healthy balanced diet so much easier.

The What's Inside Guide is supported by some of the biggest names in the industry like Cadbury, Coca-Cola Great Britain, Danone, Kellogg's, Kraft, Masterfoods, Nestle, Quaker, Ryvita, Tate & Lyle, Unilever and Walkers.

The system has gathered a lot of support from organisations associated with health in the UK, including Diabetes UK, showing how useful this scheme can be.

Commenting on the new food labelling system on behalf of Diabetes UK, Douglas Smallwood, the charity's Chief Executive, said: 'It is vital that people with diabetes and those seeking to reduce the risk of developing the condition get information about foods to help make the right choices about what to eat. The FSA has undertaken a long period of research and consultation to get a scheme that will be effective. However, voluntary labelling will only work if manufacturers adhere to these guidelines. Providing information in different formats is likely to be little better than giving no information at all, so it's really important that the food industry is consistent.'

Speaking for the British Heart Foundation, Peter Hollins, Director General, added: 'The BHF supports the FSA's approach to front of pack signpost labelling as it offers instant help to shoppers at the point of sale. We think it is important this information is provided in an easily understood, colour coded format, and from an independent source people can trust, such as the FSA.'

On behalf of the Royal College of Physicians, Professor Ian Gilmore, President, said of the system: 'Obesity and unhealthy eating are a real and serious threat to the health of individuals and the nation. The complex nature of this threat requires a clear and coherent strategy – the Royal College of Physicians welcomes the FSA's approach to front of pack labelling as a most necessary and practical element of such a strategy. We are impressed by the results of consumer research undertaken by the FSA which indicated that traffic light colours are key to helping consumers make healthier choices. Traffic lights will also undoubtedly assist health professionals when providing advice about healthier lifestyles.'

The Office of the Children's Commissioner, Professor Sir Albert Aynsley-Green, Children's Commissioner for England, also added: 'The Food Standard Agency's Traffic Light System delivers what consumers need: a simple method to explain what's contained in the foods they buy. This system would give shoppers more choice to make healthier purchases and has the potential to reduce obesity among our children and young people. We hope it will be used at the forefront of initiatives to limit young people's exposure to foods that are high in fat, salt and sugar.'

To read more, visit www.whatsinsideguide.com.

Weight loss

If you are overweight, it's likely to be due to eating the wrong foods, eating too much of them, eating meals in the wrong patterns each day and not taking enough exercise.

Approximately four out of every five people with Type 2 diabetes are overweight. It's unclear whether diabetes causes weight gain or weight gain causes diabetes – but they are linked and you tend to get the increased weight before you develop diabetes. Losing weight is the first step in treating Type 2 diabetes, but how do you know if you are overweight? There are charts available that show your optimal weight based on your height and gender. Once you have established what your ideal weight is, you can then see if you are over your ideal weight or not.

Body Mass Index (BMI)

This is a widely accepted measure of the amount of body fat in adults. The BMI gives us an indication of a person's ideal weight and makes it possible to find appropriate advice about attaining or maintaining that weight. However, a BMI measurement is not as accurate if you're an athlete or very muscular. Muscle weighs more than fat so this can push you into a higher BMI category even if you have a healthy level of body fat. It's also not accurate for women who are pregnant or breastfeeding, or people who are frail.

To calculate your BMI:

1. Work out your height in metres and multiply the figure by itself.

2. Measure your weight in kilograms.

3. Divide the weight by the height squared. This generates a number that you need to check against a chart of recommended BMIs.

For example, you might be 1.6m tall and weigh 65kg. The calculation would be: 1.6 x 1.6 = 2.56. BMI would be 65 divided by 2.56 = 25.39.

- Underweight = BMI less than 18.5

- Ideal = BMI 18.5-25

- Overweight = BMI 25-30

- Very obese = BMI 30-40

- Morbid obesity – sometimes called 'clinically severe obesity' – is defined as being 100lbs or more over ideal body weight or having a BMI of 40 or higher.

Other measurements you can do to establish if you are overweight include measuring your waist circumference. People who are an apple shape (fat around the waist) are more likely to develop heart disease and diabetes than those who are a pear shape (carrying weight around the bottom and upper thighs) or are more generally plump all over. A waist circumference greater than 80cm (32in) for women and 94cm (37in) for men indicates increased risk, while a measurement of more than 88cm (35in) for women and 102cm (40in) for men is considered worrying.

Your waist-hip ratio is also a good measurement of risk. This is the ratio of your waist circumference (the narrowest point on your abdomen) to your hip circumference (the widest point). Basically, if your waist is bigger than your hips then you really need to try to reduce your weight and increase your levels of exercise.

Losing weight while diabetic – either Type 1 or Type 2 – is a complicated affair. You should consult your diabetes team and see if any of the drugs you have been prescribed can lead to weight-gain, including insulin. You may want to consider eating less (rather than putting your doses up) in order to achieve balance.

If you are overweight by any of the standards we've looked at here then losing weight is probably one of the most important factors in reducing the impact of diabetes on your health. It should be pursued through improved diet, taking more exercise and doing blood tests to check you are not going 'too low', especially after exercise.

Talk to your diabetes team about your medication but don't let the added complication of diabetes put you off losing weight – it's the first step in managing it.

'Talk to your diabetes team about your medication but don't let the added complication of diabetes put you off losing weight – it's the first step in managing it.'

Summing Up

- If you take your diagnosis of diabetes seriously, you are going to have a different relationship with your food, but there's no reason why you can't eat a wide and interesting diet.

- Try not to let diabetes get in the way of food enjoyment, but listen to your body and learn how it reacts to certain food stuffs. Avoid high-fat and high-sugar foods (unless you need to eat some sugar to treat a hypo).

- Learn about the Glycaemic Index – it's a good tool to help with diabetes management.

- Keep eating (but not too much!). An eating disorder and diabetes is a dangerous combination.

- Read food labels – they are a great help in assessing the carbohydrate value of foods, as well as fat and sugar content. Not all labels are the same, so keep your head screwed on. Choose chocolate bars that tell you what the bar value is – it's much easier!

Chapter Six

Diabetes and Pregnancy

These are guidelines for diabetic women planning a pregnancy, or women who have previously had gestational (see below) diabetes and are contemplating another pregnancy.

Gestational diabetes

This is a form of diabetes that appears during pregnancy and then disappears after the baby is born. It affects about 4% of all pregnant women. Should your diabetes remain after the birth then it will get diagnosed as Type 1 or Type 2, and it means that the diabetes has only become apparent at the time of pregnancy but may have already been in existence.

If you have gestational diabetes, you must control your diabetes in much the same manner as someone who has diabetes all the time; however, it's not likely to involve insulin, only pills and diet.

You will need to blood test and be careful about what you eat – bad blood sugar control is bad for your baby, so you do need to look after yourself in order to look after the baby.

Diabetes and pregnancy

With more and more people being diagnosed with diabetes (affecting an estimated 3-4% of the UK population), the numbers of women with diabetes who also go through pregnancy is also increasing.

With ongoing improvements in understanding diabetes, along with more advanced medicines and accessories, the chances of a safe and successful outcome for mother and child are greater than they ever have been.

'This is a form of diabetes that appears during pregnancy and then disappears after the baby is born. It affects about 4% of all pregnant women.'

As with any pregnancy, you should only undertake it after proper consideration and consultation. More than ever, close control of your blood sugars will be required both for your own health and the health of the unborn child.

Blood testing

It will be important to undertake frequent blood testing, even if you do so already, and you will be encouraged to tighten up on your targets.

Blood sugar values should be as close to normal prior to conception to minimise risk to the developing baby. Fasting blood glucose (your morning blood test taken before you've eaten breakfast) should be around 6.0 mmols/L as often as possible. Aim for blood sugars below 8.0 mmols/L for the rest of the day. If you're familiar with adjusting your insulin doses based on frequent blood sugar tests then do so to meet your new targets.

Being pregnant will mean that your energy requirements will alter. How your body processes the food you eat and the insulin you take may mean you will have to change from your normal, pre-pregnancy patterns. However, it's likely that you will find control is actually easier to attain and maintain when you're pregnant.

Insulin

Many people with Type 1 diabetes now take two types of insulin each day (often in four or five injections) – a long-acting (or night-time) insulin which lasts over 24 hours, as well as a short-acting one taken at meal times which lasts up to three hours. One, or possibly both, will have to be adjusted and probably re-adjusted throughout the duration of the pregnancy, with your body returning to pre-pregnancy requirements after the birth.

You will be advised to do more blood tests, possibly as many as eight a day, in order to achieve the tight blood sugar control that is desired.

In the main, you will probably stay on the same types of insulin that you were already taking. Most of the insulins available in the UK have some studies related to them on their effects during pregnancy, but if you have major concerns, you can contact the insulin supplier for more information.

With your medical team:

- Be sure that you are comfortable with the obstetrician (childbirth consultant) who will be caring for you. Discuss each other's expectations about diabetes care during pregnancy before you become pregnant.

- Stay in touch with your medical team to discuss possible changes in insulins.

- Your doctor may advise using an insulin pump, especially if you have elevated blood sugar levels despite your best efforts.

If you are taking an ACE inhibitor (a drug which reduces high blood pressure) because of renal disease (protein in your urine) or hypertension (high blood pressure), your medical team will probably recommend that this be changed prior to conception to a tablet that is foetus friendly. Statins (cholesterol lowering tablets) also need to be reassessed if you are taking them.

If you do have kidney disease then you should consult with your medical team and possibly with a high-risk pregnancy specialist as there are additional increased risks to a pregnancy. The decision for a pregnancy in this circumstance should be made very carefully and in full consultation with your healthcare professionals.

Hypos

Plan to stay very active both before and during pregnancy, unless your obstetrician tells you to slow down. In fact, the more you exercise, the easier it should be to keep your blood sugar levels down.

However, you should carry a store of quick-acting carbohydrate with you at all times in order to treat a possible hypo, which may occur with less notice than usual as your body has increased energy requirements during pregnancy. In case of more extreme needs, be sure your partner and someone in the office knows how to give you a glucagon shot in the unlikely event that you get an extremely low blood sugar. That will mean keeping a GlucaGen HypoKit handy (GlucaGen HypoKits are available on prescription in the UK, but be sure those around you know where it is).

Keeping your insulin injection device, blood testing kit and source of sugar in one, easy to access place can help you gain and maintain good control. It will also ensure that you can quickly test and take any immediate action if necessary.

Always wear some form of identification that indicates you have diabetes if you can (see Medic Alert and Medipal in the help list at the end of this book).

The birth

If you have Type 1 diabetes, your medical team might encourage you to either be induced at around 38 weeks or to have a caesarean. This is because babies of a diabetic mother tend to be a little bit bigger than average and because the placenta can 'age' a little faster, sometimes contributing to a complicated birth. At this stage sometimes a 'sliding scale' of insulin solution and sugar solution are given via a drip, allowing the doctors to monitor control. However, if you're keen on doing blood tests during the birth, instead of going on a drip, you may be able to do so in consultation with the diabetes team and obstetrician.

Breast-feeding

Breast-feeding is encouraged, the only issue being the impact on your own energy requirements. Continued close monitoring of blood sugars is advised, mainly as you'll be tired and having hypos won't improve the situation at all. At this stage your blood sugar levels will not be an issue for the baby or affect the breast milk in any way. Good control will simply be a benefit for you at this time.

General health advice:

- Start folic acid supplements prior to conception if possible. Babies of mothers with diabetes are at increased risk of spina bifida. Folic acid has been shown to reduce this risk and should be started at least one month prior to conception and continued for at least the first six weeks of pregnancy.

- Talk to a dietician, especially if it's been a while since you last spoke to one. There are lots of new ideas that you might not know about, such as carbohydrate counting or Dose Adjustment for Normal Eating (DAFNE) (see page 97). Ideally, these need to have been considered prior to becoming pregnant rather than learned during pregnancy.

- Get your eyes examined. This is mainly just to be 'on the safe side' as pregnancy can affect the whole body, eyes included, and it's best to be aware of any changes in the eyes.

Printed information

Diabetes UK does a guide to pregnancy and diabetes, the latest edition has just been published. You can get a copy by calling Diabetes UK on 020 7424 1000. Other manufacturers, which make brands such as Accu-Check, Lifescan and Ascensia, have good literature on diabetes and pregnancy.

See the help list at the end of the book for further contacts.

Summing Up

- Work closely with your diabetes team before and during your pregnancy.

- Keep blood testing and hypo treatments handy at all times.

- Contact companies involved with diabetes for leaflets on pregnancy.

- Wear some diabetes ID – just in case you do end up having medical intervention.

- Enjoy your pregnancy and remember to look after yourself both during the pregnancy and after the birth.

Chapter Seven

Children with Diabetes

Almost all children diagnosed with diabetes have Type 1 (insulin dependent). That means insulin injections and blood testing on a daily basis, as well as keeping a keen eye on diet. However, due to various factors in modern day society (too much food, too little exercise, bad diet), Type 2 diabetes is now being diagnosed in obese children.

As parents, a diagnosis of diabetes in a child can feel devastating. It heralds some big and basic changes to the way the family operates and is a huge responsibility for the family and the child. Your child will need a steady, supportive hand from you for many years to come, and diabetes is likely to be a part of their life, possibly forever, or until a cure becomes available. However, it is manageable.

Brace yourself to be faced with a lot of new information and a steep learning curve, but be positive – help is at hand.

Children of different ages

Smaller children are unlikely to understand what's happening to them, whereas older children will have a better grasp of the fact that they now have a medical condition that they are now responsible for managing.

For younger children with diabetes there is the added problem that they are not necessarily old enough to describe how they are feeling, so you will have to watch their behaviour. One of the main factors that occurs is irritability, but it can be hard to tell a toddler (or teenage) tantrum from a hypo. After diagnosis, the easiest way to tell one 'wobbly' from another is to do a blood test. Your child won't like it, but you will have to assess if your child needs a dose of sugar or a bit of advice about manners!

There's no good age to be diagnosed with diabetes – it's going to be tough whenever it happens. Healthcare workers say that teenagers are either very good or very bad at controlling their diabetes. Why? Because it's a notoriously self-conscious age group. Having diabetes and continually having to do blood tests and injections, as well as being 'fussy' about food and eating times, really compounds that sense of being different at an age when you just want to fit in.

Then again, all diabetes management equipment is smaller, faster and more discreet than ever before, so diabetes management need not be as obvious as it used to be (the first blood test machines were the size of a brick).

So long as your child has his or her equipment with them, knows how to use it and can be persuaded to actually do so, then they'll be fine.

A lot of the equipment is actually quite cool, and most of their friends will get to the point when they'll want to do a blood test too 'just to see if they're okay'. It is safe to do this so long as you use a new lancet for each of the friends who volunteers to do it. Some might prove hard to get a drop of blood out of, while others will have geyzers. It's quite interesting (and amusing) to do, as your child's diabetic result might not be one to boast about if it's high, while their friends are likely to have what a diabetic might call 'a bit on the low side', but they'll see what your child is dealing with.

Type 1

Rising rates of childhood diabetes Type 1

Of the total population of people with diabetes, approximately 20,000 children under the age of 15 live with Type 1 diabetes in the UK at the moment.

The number of people with diabetes of all types is predicted to increase rapidly over the coming years. Type 1 diabetes is increasing in all age groups but particularly in under-fives. The current estimate of prevalence in the UK is one per 700 – 1,000 children, yielding a total population with Type 1 diabetes aged under 25 years in the UK of approximately 25,000. Local Authorities and NHS Primary Care Trusts (PCTs) might expect between 100 and 150 children with diabetes to live in their area. The peak age for diagnosis is between 10 and 14 years of age.

'Of the total population of people with diabetes, approximately 20,000 children under the age of 15 live with Type 1 diabetes in the UK at the moment.'

Treating Type 1 diabetes in children

By definition, Type 1 diabetes is treated with insulin injections. Part of insulin therapy is frequent blood testing and, depending on the age of the child, either you or they will have to learn how to use a blood test machine and how to do injections. At diagnosis these are the first skills that you should be instructed in.

Children tend not to be put on the same type of insulin therapy as adults, due to the fact that they do not have the same hormonal landscape and so on. Often they will be started on one or two injections a day, whereas an adult is likely to take a long-acting (or 'background') insulin injection (which lasts for 24 hours) and additional injections with each meal.

It will be during the teenage years that the therapy will be adjusted onto the adult regime. Although this sounds more arduous as it has more injections, it should give greater control, leading to greater freedom and flexibility, so it should not be sniffed at. However, it will mean that your child (or young adult by this stage) will have to carry their insulin delivery devices with them throughout the day. It's not such a big deal, but you may need to help them remember to be organised (not a major feature of most teenage lives!).

Type 2

Rising rates of childhood diabetes Type 2

Type 2 diabetes is also on the increase due to the increased proportion of obese children in the population. Data on the prevalence of Type 2 in children is scarce but figures as high as 1,400 cases in the UK have been suggested. This could mean that there will be more than 3,000 children with Type 2 diabetes in the UK by 2013.

'According to the recent NHS report "Making Every Young Person with Diabetes Matter", there could be up to 1,400 children with Type 2 diabetes in the UK.'

Treating Type 2 diabetes in children

As Type 2 diabetes in children is directly associated with poor diet and a lack of exercise, they are likely to be treated by being put on a restricted diet and encouraged to take up exercise. If the excess weight can be lost, there is a chance that they can combat the diabetes. However, chances are it will be a part of their lives from that point on.

A child diagnosed with diabetes (and their family) will be given dietary information and may also be given a blood test machine and some pills to help regulate their blood sugar.

Diabetes and school

No matter what age your child is diagnosed with diabetes, they will have to keep going to school and must be able to look after themselves. As I have mentioned before, having diabetes is a huge responsibility. You need to be organised and grown up, which is a tall order for many children. It is unfair, but not impossible to handle.

Tips on diabetes and schooling:

- You must tell the school about the diagnosis. It would be dangerous for your child if they got into trouble with their diabetes and the school did not know how to help.

- Having well-controlled diabetes will not in any way lessen your child's ability to perform well, either academically or in sports. In the main, good control is down to being diligent about blood testing, eating good food on a regular basis and generally taking good care of yourself.

- Get you and your child organised. How organised will depend very much on the age of the child and his or her medication. For younger children, the school secretary or a nominated teacher should have access to a blood test machine (or know where the child keeps it) and know how to use it. Older children (I would suggest aged eight and above, but it would depend on their ability to do this themselves) should carry a blood test machine with them, along with any medication they take and a sugar source of some sort in order to combat a low blood sugar.

'You must tell the school about the diagnosis. It would be dangerous for your child if they got into trouble with their diabetes and the school did not know how to help.'

- Tell the teacher. They'll need a basic understanding of diabetes, how to tell if your child is having a hypo and how to help them treat it. Helpful information (including factsheets) on how to manage your child's diabetes at school and what a teacher needs to know are available from Diabetes UK, JDRF (Juvenile Diabetes Research Foundation) and the IDDF (Insulin Dependent Diabetes Trust). See the help list for details.

- Tell your child's friends and their parents. You'll get used to putting this simply for them, but it's best for your child if their friends know what he or she is dealing with and about the possibility of hypos. Your child will be in their company when at school, so enlist them in helping your child. This applies at all ages and particularly through the teenage years when your child is enjoying a growing social life and maybe attending concerts, parties, etc.

When I was a kid, back in the 1970s, the school secretary kept a box of sugar cubes in her desk; if I felt 'wobbly', I'd go and ask for some. This was before blood test machines, but I was only on two injections a day (one in the morning and one in the evening) and both of those were administered at home by my mother.

Coping with diabetes at school is part of the way that a child starts to understand that they are in charge of their own wellbeing. They need to be aware of how they are feeling in terms of their diabetes – if they are thirsty, do they have high blood sugar? If they are unable to concentrate, do they have a low blood sugar? Do they need to tell someone they feel funny? Do they need to let the teacher know they need to do a blood test and maybe eat a snack in class?

This is where children come up against that horrid feeling of being different and not wanting to stand out. But they need to develop a sense of responsibility – they have to look after themselves, no matter what anyone else thinks about it. Their friends will get used to it and their teachers will be sympathetic and helpful.

Travelling with a diabetic child

If your family is going on holiday you will need to check that you have the right medication and equipment to handle your child's diabetes before you go. Take lots of spares with you just in case and remember to look after insulin by making sure bottles or cartridges can't be broken. Insulin should be kept cool but will be fine so long as it's not exposed to extremes of temperature. Always keep insulin in your hand luggage; it must not go in the hold of an airplane as it could freeze and become inactive. You might want to keep it in a safe place and let the rest of the family know where it is.

If you are not going to be with your child, be sure they know what medication to take, how to take it and when. They should be able to do a blood test on their own and understand the result. Presumably, depending on the reason for travel and the age of your child, there will be some adults involved. It would be good to tell a responsible adult that your child has diabetes and show them what the equipment is so they don't get any surprises later on.

Diabetes is getting more common – virtually everyone has heard of it – so chances are some of these adults will have come across it before and can be helpful and supportive to your child.

As a result of living with diabetes, I've designed kitbags specifically for carrying diabetes management equipment around, as travelling, even just commuting, can be stressful if you're not prepared for all eventualities regarding your diabetes. See page 85 for more information on kitbags.

Teenagers, young adults and diabetes

This age range is famous for either being very good or very bad with their control. Seeing blood test results written down or printed from a PC is not as important as knowing that the blood tests are at least being done.

The teenage years are hard – full of spots, exams and worrying about your looks – so having a medical condition is just another pressure. Try and help keep your son or daughter on the straight-and-narrow, but you will have to tread a line between being caring and being overbearing and interfering. It's your child, and their welfare ranks very highly in your life, so you may have to just get on their nerves a little while you keep an eye on them.

You will figure out the time to let them go to their hospital or GP appointments on their own, but if you're both happy to go together then that's fine. Your medical advisor won't object as it's understood that diabetes affects the whole family.

Summing Up

- Get kitted up with easy-to-use blood testing machines and a 'finger-pricker' (lancing device) that can be adjusted to suit small fingers.

- Try to get into a routine of blood testing and eating healthy meals at regular times.

- Talk to your child about what they have to deal with – ultimately, they will have to take over their diabetes themselves.

- Keep school teachers and parents of your child's friends informed. They may have to look after your child and they should be informed as to what they need to look out for.

- Contact the larger diabetes-related companies for information about children and diabetes and get a copy of 'From Tots to Teens' from Diabetes UK.

- Try to keep a diary of blood test results and make it as fun as possible to fill it in. Good results can be rewarded (not food rewards though).

- Do not punish a child for 'bad' blood test results, just look at why they may have happened – many people with diabetes get a lot of extremely varied results, the point is to try to avoid extremes of highs and lows.

- Any diabetes, but Type 1 in particular, is likely to be a life-long companion to your child, so you need to help them keep their head straight about living with the condition. Don't frighten them or let them feel they are failing – that won't help at all!

- There is a saying, 'trust in Allah but remember to tie up your camel'. In the same way, trust your teenager but keep an eye on them. It's an easy age to fall prey to cynicism or despair, leading to lousy diabetes control and possible depression. Keep taking an interest, even if they don't want you to!

Chapter Eight

Diabetes Management Equipment

Diabetes research

There is a lot of research going on into all aspects of Type 1 and Type 2 diabetes, as well as some other rare subdivisions of diabetes. Some of the research is right down to bio-chemical levels and some is to do with the make up of the human genome.

Some research looks into best practice for managing diabetes from a psychological point of view. Even with modern medical science, much of diabetes treatment and management is about human care. The role of healthcare workers in diabetes care is to guide, inform and support patients, as well as using the appropriate medications to control diabetes.

Research is, by its very nature, ongoing, so stay in touch with diabetes healthcare professionals for research updates. The Internet is a good resource for more information and you can find out a lot about current research if you are interested. Otherwise go to the leading diabetes charities for information on diabetes research in the UK: Diabetes UK, DRWF, JDRF and IDDT (see end of book for full contact details).

Don't forget that we're living in the best-ever age to have diabetes. It's not even a century since insulin was discovered and, with diabetes diagnoses on the rise, there's a lot of investment in research and making products to help diabetics manage their condition well.

'The Internet is a good resource for more information and you can find out a lot about current research if you are interested.'

Choice of equipment

In many areas of diabetes control, choice of equipment is one thing you won't be short of. What you might be short of is information on what products are available and where you can get them.

This chapter looks at some of these products; it's not an extensive list but it will contain the lead suppliers of diabetes management equipment. Bear in mind that these often change – models get upgraded or de-listed, so be aware that there may be changes after publication.

Please note that it is not possible to list the medications used to manage diabetes; in the UK the law forbids suppliers from advertising direct to patients. All drugs are supplied by prescription from GPs and other medical staff and you need to talk to them about what is available.

Where to get equipment

You'll be able to get advice and equipment from your diabetes nurse. This makes a lot of sense as they will have some familiarity with what it is you need and who to get it from. However, there's now a lot of equipment out there, so you will also need to do your own research.

- You can see many of the equipment suppliers advertising in the pages of *Balance* magazine from Diabetes UK. Otherwise, you need to go direct to suppliers (see help list).

- Bigger pharmacies might stock a choice of equipment. If you attend diabetes education days, they may include exhibitors whose products you can see and ask questions about.

- The Internet – in the UK there are a few websites that sell diabetes products. There are lots in the USA – with 20 million diabetics across America, you can see why some websites have pages and pages of products.

Blood test machines (or blood glucose meters)

There are between 30 to 40 different blood test machines available in the UK, some of which are sold in pharmacies.

You will probably be given a blood test machine if you are diagnosed with Type 1 diabetes. But if you want to search for one, first figure out what it is you are looking for in a machine – do you want a small one, one with a bigger screen, a faster one or one that you can use to download your results onto your PC? In some cases, you may find a lot of information about a product on the manufacturer's website, or you can call them if you'd like to see a brochure. There are even blood test machines that have acoustic properties, so if you are sight-impaired you can 'hear' your blood test result via a series of beeps.

Blood test machines – points to consider

- Size – how will you carry this? Do you prefer to use a smaller or a larger machine?

- Speed – most machines are pretty fast these days, but it's best to check first.

- How big does the drop of blood need to be for the machine to operate?

- Sensors – how sensitive are they? Can they cope with being handled? How big is the pot they come in and do they even come in a pot?

- Individual sensors versus barrels or drums. Some machines use a system whereby a drum is dropped into the machine and you use it up (usually 10 sensors in a drum) before having to change the barrel, which may suit some users.

- Memory capability – if you don't write your results down, a long memory might come in handy.

- Download capability – via cable or Bluetooth?

- Screen – small screen or large screen?

- Support – is there a helpline to call if you need to ask a question?

Blood test machine suppliers

ABBOTT DIABETES CARE

- Precision QID.
- Optium.
- Optium Xceed.
- Freestyle Lite.
- Freestyle Mini.
- Freestyle Freedom Lite.
- Freestyle Freedom.
- Freestyle Classic.
- Medisense G2.
- Softsense.

ACCU-CHEK (Roche)

- Aviva.
- Active.
- Compact.
- Compact Plus.

ASCENSIA (BAYER)

- Breeze.
- Contour.
- Contour II.

MENARINI

- Glucomen PC.
- Glucomen Glyco.

LIFESCAN (Johnson & Johnson)

- One Touch 2.
- One Touch Ultra Smart.
- One Touch Ultra Easy.

Lancing devices

Most lancing devices come with whichever blood test machine you opt for. Most now have a mechanism that allows you to adjust the depth the lancet goes to – a child will not need the lancet to penetrate as deep as a grown man would. One thing you may want to take into consideration is how to dispose of lancets – some of the newer ones retract so that there are no sharp bits left exposed. You could also invest in sharps bins (see page 87) and put used needles and lancets in there to see that they are safely disposed of.

Lancing device suppliers

ABBOTT DIABETES CARE

- Medisense Easy Touch.
- Freestyle Lancing Device.

ACCU-CHEK (Roche)

- Accu-Chek Softclix.
- Accu-Chek Softclix Pro.
- Accu-Chek Multiclix.

ASCENSIA (Bayer)

- Microlet.
- Microlet Vaculance.

BECTON DICKINSON

- BD Optimus.

DIAGNOSYS MEDICAL

- Gentle Draw.

LIFESCAN (Johnson & Johnson)

- One Touch UltraSoft.

MENARINI

- GlucoJet Dual.

OWEN MUMFORD

- Autolet Impression.

Insulin delivery devices

Syringes

Although not used as much these days, some people prefer syringes or have an insulin that is not supplied in insulin pen-and-cartridge form. All are made of plastic and are disposable. They come in 0.5ml to 3ml sizes and beyond.

Disposable syringe suppliers

- BD (Becton Dickinson).

- BD Micro-Fine Insulin Syringe.
- Micro-Fine Pen Needle.

Insulin pens

These are likely to be dictated by the insulin you are on, which will be decided by you and your doctor. Novo insulins are delivered by Novopens. Humulin insulin from Eli Lilly gets delivered via a Humapen. These use disposable needles (see overleaf). Some pens are pre-filled which means you don't need to get insulin in cartridges but get a pre-filled pen that you dispose of when finished. You will still need to replace the needles.

Insulin pen suppliers

- Novo Nordisk (the Novopen range).
- Eli Lilly (the Humapen range).
- Owen Mumford (the Autolet range).

Insulin pumps

What are they?

Pumps are a relatively old idea, but interest in them dwindled, mainly as it was considered that there would be a cure for diabetes so there was no need to pursue pump technology. A more recent resurgence of pump therapy is due to the fact that there is no immediate cure in sight and there are now a lot more diabetics. It's also seen as a great tool for those who want to get very close control as the pump is a subtle insulin deliverer.

How does it work?

An insulin pump has a reservoir in it where the insulin is stored and delivered on a continuous basis 24-hours a day. This is called the basal rate and the amount can be varied so that you get slightly more per hour in the mornings and less in the afternoons, if that is what your personal profile requires. On top of that, you could give yourself a 'bolus' (a dose) when required, for example at meal times. The bolus would be based on your estimate of your food in terms of carbohydrate value and GI, as well as what you are about to do in terms of exercise.

The pump is attached to the body via a thin tube which is connected by an infusion set. This is not something that is surgically implanted – you put the infusion set in by yourself, changing the set every three days.

You still need to blood test. There is ongoing research into continuous blood testing, much done by the makers of insulin pumps, but it's not cheap and it's not that reliable yet.

How do I get one?

Well, this is the hard bit. These are expensive items – you can buy one yourself but they cost about £2,500, and a year's supply of the additional items that you need will cost about another £500.

Only a few NHS trusts currently offer them, but that's no reason not to ask. You are more likely to get a pump if you are a Type 1 diabetic and a frequent blood tester, have an idea about carbohydrate counting and are prepared to get used to using the pump and having it attached.

Insulin pump suppliers

- Accu-chek (the Spirit insulin pump).
- Medtronic (the Paradigm range of pumps).
- Lifescan (Johnson & Johnson – the Animus pump).

Needles

With needles often you will use the same needles produced by the manufacturer of your insulin pen. The main variation in needles is the length of the needle and, in some cases, the width of the needle too. The disposable needles screw onto the insulin pen.

It's a good idea to dial in a few units of insulin to see if everything is working before you actually give yourself a dose. It's recommended that you change the needle for each injection, but many diabetics use a needle for at least one whole day (and many just keep using it until it goes blunt enough to hurt and therefore warrant changing it).

Needle suppliers

- BD (Becton Dickinson).
- Novo Nordisk, Novofine needles.
- Owen Mumford (see Medical Shop), Unifine Pentips.

Other products

Kitbags and carriers

As a diabetic you need to carry around a whole bunch of stuff with you in order to manage your condition. Make it easier on yourself and get organised. Get a bag that you like and pack it full of the stuff you need to have with you.

For a Type 1 diabetic you are likely to need:

- Blood test machine.
- Lancing device.
- Tub of sensors.
- Spare lancets.
- Spare sensors.
- Diary and pen.
- Insulin pen with needle and cartridge.
- Spare needles.
- Spare cartridge.

'As a diabetic you need to carry around a whole bunch of stuff with you in order to manage your condition. Make it easier on yourself and get organised. Get a bag that you like and pack it full of the stuff you need to have with you.'

- Hypo treatment.

Diabetes bags and carry-case suppliers

- Desang – specialises in fitting monitoring and medicating diabetes management equipment in specially designed kitbags.

- Frio – specialises in keeping insulin cool and protected.

- Medicool.

- Medipak.

Identification products

A great idea, and some of them aren't that bad! Medic Alert is a charity but you pay membership for them to keep your details on their database. If you wear one of their tags and get into trouble (for example, you are found unconscious) anyone tending to you will be able to ring in and check your medical condition and medications. Doctors and nurses should be on the look out for these tags – they are quite well-known.

ID tag suppliers

- Medipal – looks like a credit-card but with medical information on it.

- Medic Alert – range of bracelets and necklaces with a phone number on. The number can be called and relevant medical history (for example, if you have Type 1 or Type 2 diabetes, what your medication is, etc) is told to the person trying to help you.

Sharps bins

These are specific bins into which you put used needles, lancets and other bits and bobs you would like to be kept safely out of the way until disposing of them. These are labelled so that refuse collectors also know what they are dealing with – these bins and their contents ought to be incinerated. See help list for details of how to obtain these.

Impotence products

Due to the fact that diabetes can cause vascular damage, it's possible that men with diabetes could develop erectile dysfunction and may require information on impotence products. See help list for contact details.

For hypo treatments, see chapter 4.

Summing Up

- There's a lot of diabetes management equipment out there, but it's not that easy to find. Get a copy of Diabetes UK's publication, *Balance*, which has a lot of relevant advertisers in it.

- Find kit that you like to use. Most of us don't like pricking our fingers, but we'll do it more often if we think we've found a lancing device that does not hurt much – likewise with injections. Shop around and ask around – you may find that someone has the product that's right for you.

- Don't forget the best bit of kit you've got is your head – keep yourself informed about your condition to help you make the best of what is available to you.

- Go direct to manufacturers for product information packs and leaflets on aspects of living with diabetes. There's a lot of good information available to those who ask!

Chapter Nine

Diabetes Complications

Diabetes is a medical condition that you have to take seriously. You can live a good life with it, but it does impose a discipline and you are better off working with it rather than fighting against it. The only person who will get damaged if you don't 'play by the rules' is you (and possibly those who care about you). Consider it a house-guest – one you did not invite to stay, but now they're here you might as well get along with them.

The Diabetes Control and Complications Trial (DCCT) was a 10-year study undertaken from 1983 to 1993 (funded by the National Institute of Diabetes and Digestive and Kidney Diseases) in order to assess the effects of intensive therapy on the long-term complications of diabetes. The study very clearly showed that intensive management (i.e. close control) of insulin-dependent diabetes prevents or slows the development of the long-term complications of diabetes (eye, kidney and nerve damage).

If you don't manage to control your diabetes you are running the considerable risk of contracting what are referred to as 'diabetes complications', some of which we look at here.

The following information is a broad summary of the main conditions (or complications) that are associated with diabetes, especially if it is not well-controlled.

Diabetic retinopathy

What is it?

- This is damage to the back of the eye (the retina) caused by diabetes.
- Regularly having high blood sugars will contribute to this condition.

- It can be treated with laser therapy, up to a point.

Diabetes is the leading cause of blindness in adults of working age in the western world. That is a sobering statistic and shows you why you should make every effort to control your diabetes and get your eyes checked at least annually.

'Diabetes is the leading cause of blindness in adults of working age in the western world. That is a sobering statistic and shows you why you should make every effort to control your diabetes and get your eyes checked at least annually.'

What can you do?

- You are entitled to free eye tests if you have diabetes. Make sure you get regular check-ups with your optician; they will be able to spot if there are any diabetic changes happening in your eyes.

- More and more PCTs (NHS Primary Care Trusts) are offering people with diabetes a special eye test once a year where digital photos are taken of the backs of your eyes in order to keep track of the eye's health.

According to Diabetes UK, 'All patients over 12 should be screened annually by their local quality controlled diabetic retinopathy screening service. You should automatically be sent an invitation to have your eyes screened by this service. If you don't, then ask your GP or diabetes clinic about the screening service in your area. If no service is offered in your area, Diabetes UK can support you to lobby your local health provider. It is still important to have annual examinations of the back of your eye and you should ask your GP or diabetes team to refer you or recommend a local service which offers retinal screening to an appropriate standard.'

So, keep a close eye on those eyes of yours and make sure you get regular check-ups. Any high street opticians ought to be able to give you a quick once-over if you do have concerns.

Should you end up with a diagnosis of retinopathy, you are likely to be put forward for laser treatment. The laser treatment cauterises (literally 'burns' in order to seal) new blood vessels which the eye has grown in order to overcome the effects of damage to the original blood vessels in the eye. This is relatively painless and can be effective in keeping the effects of retinopathy at bay, but you will need to continue to do your part in trying to control your blood sugar levels.

Diabetic neuropathy

What is it?

This is nerve damage caused by elevated blood sugars. It tends to happen in the extremities of the body – the fingers and, more particularly, the toes.

When damage occurs, the blood vessels feeding nutrients to the nerves in your hands and feet can become deprived, which stops the nerves operating effectively. This may not be something that you notice; some people wind up with tingling and other sensations, so it may be that you get nerve damage and don't know about it. You are in no pain and, as far as you are aware, you're fine.

If the nerve is damaged it may not report pain back up to the brain, so infection can set in to a cut or abrasion without you feeling it. Use your eyes to look for any red spots and seek advice if you do find any. Make pampering your feet part of your body maintenance and enjoy it! Feet are fab and we don't appreciate them enough.

What can you do?

Look after those blood sugar levels! The main other thing you should do is check your feet for damage that you may not have actually felt (look for redness, cracking or cuts). Take a few minutes to give them a good look once a week or so.

If damage has occurred and you are not checking your feet, you can scrape your foot or stand on something and, because you can't feel it, it could lead to an infection. That infection, if not noticed and treated, could in the worst-case scenario lead to gangrene and amputation. So check your feet regularly and wear slippers when indoors!

There are gels and creams that can be used to help keep foot skin soft and supple, such as Flexitol, Heel Balm and Hypogeen Foot Cream. See www.foot. com for more information. This useful and detailed American site includes a section on 'the diabetic foot.'

Diabetic neuropathy can also affect the hands, but they're a little easier to see. If you start to get regular bouts of pins and needles you should mention this to your healthcare worker.

There's a slightly higher incidence of certain other medical conditions that seem to link themselves to diabetes, particularly in arms and hands, such as frozen shoulder, Carpal Tunnel Syndrome and Dupuytren's Contracture. These need to be addressed by specialists but your diabetes team can refer you if they think it's necessary.

Frozen shoulders often go away after time, and Carpel Tunnel Syndrome can be treated. To avoid extra strain on yourself you can look into how to avert the syndrome, which is associated particularly with repetitive activities like typing. Learning good techniques can lessen the impact and might avoid the need for surgery.

Diabetic nephropathy

Also known as diabetic kidney disease, diabetic nephropathy is a complication of diabetes. If you have this condition your kidney loses its ability to function properly. The condition is characterised by high protein levels in the urine, which is why your doctor may occasionally ask you to do a urine (or microalbuminuria) test.

Kidneys are made of hundreds of thousands of units called nephrons. Each nephron has a cluster of blood vessels called a glomerulus. The glomerulus filters blood and forms urine, which drains down into the ureter.

The earliest detectable change in the course of diabetic nephropathy is a thickening in the glomerulus. At this stage, the kidney may start allowing more albumin (protein) in the urine than normal, and this can be detected by sensitive tests for albumin. This stage is called microalbuminuria (micro refers to the small amounts of albumin).

As diabetic nephropathy progresses, increasing numbers of glomeruli are destroyed. The amount of albumin being excreted in the urine increases and may be detected by ordinary urinalysis techniques. At this point, a kidney biopsy clearly shows diabetic nephropathy.

Protein may appear in the urine for five to 10 years before other symptoms develop; for example, high blood pressure often accompanies diabetic nephropathy. Over time, the kidney's ability to function starts to decline and diabetic nephropathy may eventually lead to chronic kidney failure. This continues to progress toward end-stage kidney disease, often within two to six years after the appearance of high protein in the urine (proteinuria).

People with both Type 1 and Type 2 diabetes are at risk, the risk being higher if blood-glucose levels are poorly controlled. However, once nephropathy develops, the greatest rate of progression is seen in patients with poor control of their blood pressure.

Diabetic nephropathy generally goes along with other diabetes complications, including hypertension, retinopathy and blood vessel changes, although these may not be obvious during the early stages of nephropathy.

Early stage diabetic nephropathy has no symptoms. Symptoms develop late in the disease and may be a result of kidney failure or eliminating high amounts of protein in the urine.

Diabetic nephropathy symptoms may include:

- Fatigue.
- Foamy appearance or excessive frothing of the urine.
- Frequent hiccups.
- General ill feeling.
- Generalised itching.
- Headache.
- Nausea and vomiting.
- Poor appetite.
- Swelling of the legs.
- Swelling, usually around the eyes in the mornings. General body swelling may occur with late-stage disease.
- Unintentional weight gain (from fluid build up).

'Diabetic nephropathy generally goes along with other diabetes complications, including hypertension, retinopathy and blood vessel changes, although these may not be obvious during the early stages of nephropathy.'

Diabetes and depression

Depression is not necessarily associated with diabetes, but you should be aware that as someone living with a long-term chronic condition you may find yourself feeling like you can't cope.

Diabetes is a huge responsibility – you have to take care of your health in ways that most people have the luxury of taking for granted. You have to understand your medication, think about your diet and keep an eye on your weight. Your blood sugars may be hard to control or you might fear the onset of diabetes complications.

With Type 1 diabetes (and some cases of Type 2 diabetes) you have to do regular blood tests and regular injections. It's a high-maintenance regime and it can feel like a real burden.

'If you are feeling overwhelmed, take heart that there is help available. Ask your GP or other medical personnel who work with you for help. They will be able to point you in the right direction.'

Requiring access to diabetes management equipment like a blood test machine (plus lancing device and tub of sensors), as well as pills or insulin pens (with spare insulin and needles), might make you feel uneasy about going out and about. The prospect of having an unexpected hypo might also keep you keen on staying at home or thinking that 'running a bit high' is okay because it means you will avoid hypos. It's not a good idea though because it's the high sugars that cause the damage.

Try to get organised by putting everything you need in one bag (there are diabetes bags for this purpose, or use a pencil case or wash bag) and include a sugar source in there as well. That way, you will be safe to go out and about anywhere. Try to write down your blood test results – if you can't then just make sure you do blood tests. It's better than not blood testing at all!

Laura Plunkett, a mother of a child with diabetes, says: 'As with any chronic disease, you have to keep generating renewed enthusiasm; otherwise, you settle into ruts without noticing how lax you've become.'

If you are feeling overwhelmed, take heart that there is help available. Ask your GP or other medical personnel who work with you for help. They will be able to point you in the right direction.

Feeling a sense of hopelessness and despair are features of depression, along with not wanting to talk about it. However, recognise these as symptoms of depression, not of diabetes, and ask for help. Diabetes has its ups and downs, and it's quite common for people with diabetes to feel depressed from time to time. This may be aggravated by variations in your blood sugar levels or by the stress of dealing with your diabetes every day.

If you think you are suffering from 'diabetes burnout', talk to your diabetes nurse, your partner, a close friend or try a support group. If things don't seem to be getting better, tell your doctor – they can advise you on any appropriate treatment or counselling if necessary.

Summing Up

- Prevention is not only better than a cure, there may not be a cure for some complications, so know your rights and make sure your diabetes team see you at least three times a year, have an annual medical and get your eyes checked at least annually.

- If you are worried about any aspect of your health which may be related to your diabetes, call your healthcare professional for advice.

- Try not to worry. If you're looking after yourself then complications are not inevitable.

- Diabetes can be a really big deal, but we've all got lives to live as well as looking after our diabetes. If it all feels like it's getting too much, talk. There is help available, but you may need to ask for it.

Chapter Ten

Additional Information

Educational programmes

Depending on whether you're newly diagnosed or are in fact a little 'long in the tooth' when it comes to your diabetes, you may be aware of the changing and enlarging vocabulary of diabetes management.

DAFNE

DAFNE stands for Dose Adjustment for Normal Eating. DAFNE is a way of managing Type 1 diabetes and provides people with the skills necessary to estimate the carbohydrate in each meal and to inject the right dose of insulin. It helps show people how they can fit diabetes into their lifestyle, rather than having to radically change their lifestyle to fit in with their diabetes.

Proving that it's not only what you do but it's the way that you do it, it's been established that DAFNE can help people with diabetes lead more flexible (or 'normal') lives and improve blood glucose control. The DAFNE approach, which is still being studied by researchers throughout the UK, is based on an educational programme designed by the late Dr. Michael Berger in Dusseldorf, Germany.

I've been on it myself (I am a DAFNE graduate of some years standing!) and I've also read about its success rate. The DAFNE course involves attending a five-day training course (9am to 5pm, Monday to Friday), which sounds like – and is – a huge commitment. When I went on the course, I'd had Type 1 diabetes for 30 years. Having been taught to 'count carbs' since childhood, not everything on the course was new, but what I learnt was up-to-date and very reassuring for someone who had wearied of the constant judging of food amounts and insulin doses. I've heard it referred to as 'teaching old dogs new tricks' as the course is often offered to old-timers like myself, but it's a great basis for anyone handling an insulin regime.

The structured teaching programme is delivered to groups of six to eight participants and covers topics including carbohydrate estimation, counting carbohydrates, blood glucose monitoring, insulin regimens, hypos, illness and exercise. You will practise the skills of carbohydrate estimation and insulin adjustment under the supervision of DAFNE-trained nurses and dieticians. Most of the training is built around group work, sharing and comparing experiences with other people with Type 1 diabetes.

Initially I'd not been too impressed with having to take a week off work and sit in a room with other diabetics, but it was a very rewarding experience, giving me a real boost of confidence that I was, in the main, doing things right and that I was not alone with the problems of control that I faced.

According to a press release from Diabetes UK, published in November 2005, 'DAFNE has undergone a Randomised Control Trial, the results of which showed improved glycaemic control (lower HbA1c) without any increase in severe hypoglycaemia, along with significant improvement to quality of life and treatment satisfaction. A training programme has been developed to train doctors and diabetes educators so they can deliver the DAFNE model. The programme currently meets all the NICE criteria for structured education programmes for people with diabetes.'

Ask your diabetes team about access to this course in your area. Visit www.dafne.uk.com for more information.

DESMOND

DESMOND stands for Diabetes Education and Self Management for Ongoing and Newly Diagnosed. Don't worry about remembering this – even the medical staff you know might struggle to remember what it stands for!

'DESMOND stands for Diabetes Education and Self Management for Ongoing and Newly Diagnosed. This is also a structured group education programme, but it's mainly for people with Type 2 diabetes.'

This is also a structured group education programme, but it's mainly for people with Type 2 diabetes. Diabetes specialists use it to provide a structured education about diabetes management (healthy diet choices, blood testing and weight management advice) with its clinical management (the pills and even insulin).

Ask your diabetes team about access to this course in your area. Visit www.desmond-project.org.uk for further information.

Driving and diabetes

As there is a risk of hypoglycaemia (hypo) if your diabetes is treated with insulin or with certain diabetes tablets, you should do a blood test before you undertake any car journey as the driver. If you are not sure if your tablets can cause a hypo, discuss this with your healthcare team.

Having a hypo while you are in charge of a motor vehicle can be fatal, not only for you, but for others as well. Whether driving or not, you should always carry some form of glucose with you in your pocket or handbag, and always be sure to have a hypo treatment handy in the car.

The following information was taken from an information sheet published by Diabetes UK in July 2006 and is still valid: 'If you have diabetes that is treated with insulin you must, by law, inform the Driver and Vehicle Licensing Agency (DVLA) as soon as possible after you have been diagnosed. If you have diabetes that is treated with tablets as well as another relevant condition or complication, you must also, by law, inform the DVLA.

'After you have filled in and returned your application form, if you are treated with insulin you will be sent another form (called "Diabetic 1") asking for more information and for the name and address of your GP and/or hospital doctor. You will also be asked to fill in a consent form so that the DVLA can approach your doctor, or other relevant healthcare professional, directly if necessary.

'This form must be completed if your diabetes is treated with insulin. This procedure does not mean that you will be refused a driving licence. The DVLA just needs to be sure that every licensed driver is going to be safe on the road. So long as your diabetes is well-controlled and you have no complications that might impair your safety as a driver – and your doctor confirms this if asked – there is no reason why you should not be issued with a licence. It is important that you answer the questions honestly.

'If you are treated with tablets, the DVLA will send you a letter. This explains that you must re-notify them if your condition or treatment changes (for example, if you have to go onto insulin or if you start to have hypos) or if you develop any of the complications of diabetes. However, they will not normally ask any further questions about your diabetes at this time and you will normally be allowed to keep your "til 70" licence.

'Restricted licences: if you take insulin you will be issued with a licence for one, two or three years. Just before the expiry date you will receive a reminder to renew and you will be asked to return your current licence. You will also be sent another "Diabetic 1" form to confirm your medical condition...

'If you are treated with tablets or diet alone you may be issued with a "til 70" licence. If you are treated by diet alone you will be issued with a "til 70" licence. However, you should inform the DVLA if you develop any complications as a result of your diabetes or if you require treatment with insulin. When this licence expires you will need to renew it every one to three years, just like other people in the UK who are over 70 years old...Provisional licences are restricted to one, two or three years only if your diabetes is treated with insulin.

'If you do have a hypoglycaemic episode at the wheel, you may be charged with driving under the influence of a drug, insulin, driving without due care and attention, or dangerous driving. Therefore, it is essential that you check your blood glucose levels to make sure this does not happen.'

Contact details

DVLA Drivers enquiries: 08:00 – 20:30 Monday to Friday and 08:00 – 17.30 on Saturday. Tel: 0870 240 0009.

Address: Drivers Customer Services (DCS) Correspondence Team, DVLA, Swansea, SA6 7JL (to avoid delay with written enquiries it is important to use the correct postcode). Email: drivers.dvla@gtnet.gov.uk.

Travelling with diabetes

Travelling, overnight stays and short trips should not cause any real anxieties (unless the diabetic is a young child). For adults, short trips are easy enough. You will need to take all your normal stuff with you and might need to remember to take your long-acting insulin as well.

Check your supplies before you go – do you have enough blood test sensors to last you? What about insulin and hypo treatment (just in case)?

Longer trips and overseas travel need a bit more forethought and planning. Put a date in your diary to check all your supplies two weeks before you go and to get anything extra you may need from your GP.

With security now such an issue, it's good to keep your diabetes kit and medication in one place so you can easily access it and, if required, show it at customs. As diabetes is now quite common you should not have any issues with this in the UK, USA and many Western countries.

One thing not to forget is that you should definitely keep your insulin in your hand luggage. It must not go in the hold of an airplane as it may freeze, making it inactive. It's also good practice to keep your medications with you so they are not lost. The last thing you need is medical equipment going missing! Keep it with you, keep it safe, don't let it get too hot or cold and you'll be fine.

Other tips for travelling overseas

- Contact Diabetes UK to see if they have a factsheet on the country you are visiting.

- Get the address of the British Consulate in the country you are visiting and have that handy in case you need advice from people who speak your language and know the local culture.

- If you're travelling with people whom you do not know, it is wise to tell them you have diabetes. It's not fair on them if you're suddenly taken ill and they don't know what to do to help you!

- Keep a hypo treatment handy at all times – new cultures and new foods may well lead to unexpected high or low sugars.

■ If you are travelling to very hot climates you will need to keep your insulin cool. See below for more information.

Keeping insulin cool

The main information on how you need to look after your insulin supplies will come from the makers of the insulin itself. Each bottle or box of cartridges has an information sheet in it. You can also check with your diabetes nurse and GP, but if you use some common sense and keep your insulin away from extremes of temperature, you should be okay. When it's not in use (unopened and not in an insulin pen), it should be kept in a fridge. If it's in use – an open bottle of insulin or a cartridge already loaded into a pen or in an insulin pump – the insulin should be fine at room temperature for several weeks.

If you think it necessary, there are specialist bags and carry cases that keep insulin cool. There are even mini-fridges that you can plug into the car to keep insulin cool if you are travelling in very hot countries.

Travel resources

An excellent diabetes and travel website is www.diabetes-travel.co.uk/home.htm. Here you can find information on preparation, getting to your destination, bureaucracy, travelling with insulin, insulin pumps, diet and alcohol, time zones and keeping well – the list goes on! The site is supported by the Western General Hospital Trust Edinburgh and Diabetes UK Edinburgh Branch.

A diabetic traveller's checklist

Anyone travelling anywhere with diabetes, especially when travelling overseas, should have a note with them from their doctor saying that they have diabetes and are on medication. A pump user may need an additional letter from their hospital or clinic saying that they are diabetic and on a pump.

I know I'm repeating myself, but do not forget that insulin cannot go in the hold as it may freeze, which can deactivate it. It's best to carry all your medication and diabetes management equipment with you in your hand luggage where you can also keep an eye on it.

'Anyone travelling anywhere with diabetes, especially when travelling overseas, should have a note with them from their doctor saying that they have diabetes and are on medication.'

For Type 2:

If you have a blood test machine you may wish to take it with you, along with your medications.

For injectors:

- Blood test machine.
- Lancing device.
- Blood test sensors.
- Insulin cartridges.
- Insulin pens (long-acting and short-acting).
- Needles.
- Hypo treatment.

For pump users:

- Reservoirs.
- Infusion sets.
- Infusion set inserter.
- Bottles of insulin.
- Batteries for pump.
- Blood test machine.
- Lancing device.
- Blood test sensors.
- Hypo treatment.

You may also want to take spare items on trips:

- Spare blood test machine.
- Spare sensors.
- Spare insulin.
- Spare insulin pen.
- Spare needles.
- Spare hypo treatment.
- Spare food that you are familiar with (check you're allowed to take it to the country you're travelling to as there may be restrictions).

Before you go, double-check that you have spare insulin, sensors and batteries (for pump users).

Meeting your doctor

Your medical team should be working with you to provide information, support and guidance as you are the one who will be looking after yourself on a day-to-day basis. When you are newly diagnosed it's a shock and there is a lot of information to take on board.

Make an effort to take a note of who you have seen and to understand their role. You are likely to initially see your GP who may also have a practice nurse specialising in diabetes, or perhaps one of the doctors runs special clinics. Many people with Type 1 diabetes may be referred to a diabetes clinic held in a local hospital.

It's worth getting into the habit of doing the following in order to make best use of your appointments:

- Write down any questions you have before you go to your appointment so you don't forget them.
- Take your blood test results with you and expect to have them looked at and discussed.

- Keep a diary that shows your appointments and medication (what drugs, what doses and when to take them) so you have a record that you can refer to if necessary.

- There's no such thing as a dumb question, so go ahead and ask whatever you need to until you understand the situation.

- GPs are obliged to let you have blood test sensors – do not let them fob you off with some short-term idea that sensors are expensive. Prevention of complications comes though good control. The cost of a few pots of blood test sensors now more than compensate for the cost of dialysis. You should not need to explain this to your GP, but if you are having problems getting the number of strips you think you need, call the Diabetes UK helpline for advice.

Please don't be shy – ask questions and don't expect that everything will just be fine. If someone is meant to contact you and they don't, pick up the phone and try to contact them yourself. Remember the NHS is having to cope with many more diagnoses. Ask to be referred to specialist centres if they are available and keep on top of things like your HbA1c test and other annual tests. Talk to Diabetes UK if you have concerns about your care.

Healthcare professionals are busy people and you need to look at this as a partnership – so do your bit to make the relationship work. Be pushy, but polite!

Medical Exemption Certificates (Medex)

The Authority's Medical Exemption Issue Office issues Medical Exemption Certificates on behalf of the Department of Health to patients who suffer from diabetes (unless you are treated by diet alone in which case you do not qualify for an exemption certificate). These certificates exempt you from prescription charges.

Medical Exemption Certificates are given to people resident in England. If you are resident outside England, the action you need to take to apply for a Medical Exemption Certificate depends upon the country you are resident in.

For further information call 0845 601 8076 or write to: NHS Business Services Authority, Patient Services, Medical Exemption, Newcastle upon Tyne, NE2 1ZL.

What to do when you're ill

Having diabetes does not shield you from all the other ailments people are prone to, but, once diagnosed, try not to blame everything that happens to you on diabetes. It's an added strain on your overall system but you can have a long, active and healthy life nonetheless.

'Having diabetes does not shield you from all the other ailments people are prone to, but, once diagnosed, try not to blame everything that happens to you on diabetes.'

Whatever medication you are on, you will still need to take this no matter how ill you feel. In general, if your body is fighting infection, your blood sugars are likely to rise. Looking after your diabetes when you are ill can be very tricky – you may not want to eat, you may not be able to get out of bed even, but you must keep doing your blood tests and taking your medication. It's also a good idea to keep track of your blood test results in case you need to talk them over with a GP or nurse.

If your sugars are high and are staying there, you should call your diabetes team for advice. If you are still worried, call your local hospital – you may need to go in and be seen by a doctor. If you live alone, try to tell someone that you're not well so that they can check on you.

Some illnesses, especially the ones that induce vomiting, are particularly difficult to handle. You may need to get an injection that stops the vomiting, which might involve a trip to the local hospital.

Ketoacidosis

Diabetic ketoacidosis, or DKA, is the medical term for the condition you end up with if you have a sustained high blood sugar. For more information see page 44.

Thrush

Having high blood sugars makes your already warm, wet body a very attractive home for some bacteria. As a result, thrush is often a symptom of diabetes. Advice from www.womenshealthlondon.org says: 'Diabetic women also tend to have high sugar levels in their urine, and this may contribute to thrush by feeding yeast in the genital area just outside of the vagina. Certain foods may have an impact on thrush. Some practitioners believe sugar, dairy products, coffee, tea and wine contribute to thrush by increasing urinary sugar. If your body's immune system is run down due to stress, illness, poor nutrition, HIV, fatigue or serious injury, you may be more vulnerable to thrush. This is because your body is less able to keep the infection at bay.

'A full bacteriological screen will rule out any other infections that may have similar symptoms to thrush. Thrush is caused by a fungus (candida) and is therefore treated with antifungal drugs. Treatments can be bought over the counter at a chemist, but they may be cheaper (or free) if you get them by prescription. There is also a range of alternative or complementary treatments for thrush. Not all of these treatments are supported by research, but many women find them useful. Complementary treatments tend to be most effective when used as soon as you begin to notice the symptoms of thrush.'

Essentially, we're back to the same advice: if you can keep your blood sugars under control, you ought to be able to keep thrush under control. It's important to know that the presence of thrush may be solely a result of diabetes and not sexually transmitted. If you do get thrush you will need to address it – if left alone it will be very uncomfortable and could lead to a urinary tract infection that can end up lodged in your kidneys.

You can also buy special washing products that are more pH friendly for delicate areas, which can help reduce your chances of a repeat attack. I'd also recommend that you eat yoghurt regularly as this seems to help keep the body's internal 'flora and fauna' of the bacterial world healthy so it does not impose on your day-to-day life.

Frozen shoulder

For reasons that are not entirely clear, people with diabetes have a slightly higher tendency to get frozen shoulders than the rest of the population. This is a condition where the shoulder socket loses its flexibility. In about 50% of the cases, a frozen shoulder will simply loosen back up by itself over time, but it can also take years. In other cases, you may need to have an operation where the shoulder is manipulated to break the adhesions causing the immobility.

Dupuytren's Contracture

Pronounced 'doo-pa-trens', Dupuytren's Contracture is a benign condition which causes a tightening of the flesh beneath the skin of the palm and can result in permanently bent fingers. (There are other reasons for people to develop bent fingers, including arthritis, trigger finger, the after effects of injury or Reflex Sympathetic Dystrophy, but these conditions are not Dupuytren's disease and are treated differently.)

Eye care (dry eyes)

One of the early indications of diabetes can be blurred vision. This is usually a sign of high blood sugars and should go away after diagnosis and medication is started. You may find that if you wear contact lenses your eyes may need extra moisture as diabetics tend to have dry eyes. Eye drops should be helpful, but it may mean that you have to revert back to wearing glasses. Be very vigilant with contact lenses in terms of keeping them clean because, as a diabetic, you may be more susceptible to eye infections.

As just explained, people with diabetes can tend to get dry eyes. Dry eye is characterised by dryness, burning or sandy-gritty irritation in the eyes that gets worse as the day goes on. This is a result of decreased corneal sensation or relative numbness of the surface of the eye. This relative numbness of the surface of the eye has also been associated with diabetic retinopathy (eye damage).

What is dry eye and what causes it?

An eye becomes dry when the tears lose water and become too salty. Just like when you throw salt on a wound, when your tears become too salty they cause stinging and burning of the eye surface. As the eyes become drier this becomes a sandy-gritty irritation of the eyes.

Many people choose to treat dry eyes with eye drops which will provide temporary relief of dry eye (but the dry eye itself will not get better). These include Optrex, Systane and various other drops which you can buy over the counter at any pharmacy. There is also Lacri-Lube from Allergan which is an ointment best applied at night as it can make vision blurry. Also Gel Tears or Liquivisc may help. You can also improve your intake of Omega-3s (Essential Fatty Acids) in your diet, which should help address dry eye.

See the Good Hope Hospital website at www.goodhope.org.uk where there is a downloadable leaflet about dry eyes. For information on diabetic retinopathy, see page 89.

Insomnia

Having diabetes can be a real weight on your mind at the best of times, but at night everything can seem worse. You may also have anxieties about how your control is while you are asleep. First, understand that you are not alone – everyone with diabetes has this anxiety and you'll get used to living with it. The way to avert this anxiety is to gain confidence that you are on the right medication, the right doses at the right time and that you have a good idea of what you are eating and how it will affect your blood sugars.

You could also get into the habit of having a blood test about half an hour before you go to bed so that you can address either a low or high blood test, thus avoiding the need to sort it out later in the night. Having a blood test machine near your bed is also helpful. If you wake in the night you can do a test if you think that it's a high or low blood sugar keeping you awake. It's also good to have a spare blood test meter at home should your other one be lost.

There are monitors being developed which can be programmed to give an alarm if your body is showing signs of going into hypo while you are asleep (raised heart rate, sweating).

If you continue to have problems sleeping, talk to your doctor or diabetes team.

Operations

If you have to have an operation you will need to discuss your diabetes care with whichever doctors you are dealing with. How your diabetes is handled within the hospital will vary from authority to authority – some are happy for you to continue to do blood tests and do your own injections. Others (and it will depend on the operation you are having) may want to handle your diabetes via a 'sliding scale'.

With this you'll have a drip of insulin solution going into one arm and a drip of sugar solution going into the other. The idea is that these balance each other out, giving you a steady blood sugar, especially if you are nil by mouth in anticipation of your operation.

Some operations which would be handled by Outpatients for non-diabetics may require an overnight stay for a diabetic. Take your medications, blood test machinery as well as some food and a hypo treatment with you so you have it all at hand should you need it.

Summing Up

- Be honest about your condition when it comes to jobs and driving licences. It's in your best interests as well.

- If driving, do a blood test before you set off. Make sure you have a blood test machine with you; if not in a bag that you take with you everywhere then in the glove compartment, along with a hypo treatment. You may get stuck in serious traffic, so be prepared.

- If you have concerns about any issues to do with living with diabetes, contact Diabetes UK's careline for advice.

- DAFNE and DESMOND are here to help – make at least one of them your friend!

- Your doctor is your partner in your diabetes care, so work on that relationship. Go prepared to your consultations and don't be afraid to ask questions about all aspects of your healthcare.

- When travelling, keep all your kit and medication in your hand luggage – you don't want it to be lost in transit. Insulin must not go in the hold of a plane as it can freeze and become inactive.

'Your doctor is your partner in your diabetes care, so work on that relationship. Go prepared to your consultations and don't be afraid to ask questions about all aspects of your healthcare.'

Diabetes Glossary

Ace inhibitors

Drugs used to help reduce high blood pressure, which is common in people who also have Type 2 diabetes.

Blood test machines

Small portable devices which can be used to give you a reading of your current blood sugar level (also called blood glucose), providing a useful insight into your state of diabetes control.

Blood test strip (blood test sensors)

Used in blood test machines, this is where a drop of blood is placed when it's already inserted into a blood test machine, resulting in a blood sugar reading. The aim is to have a reading in the 'normal' range of 4.0 mmols/L to 8.0 mmols/L.

Body Mass Index (BMI)

This is a formula which assesses whether you are overweight, taking into account your weight and height.

Carbohydrates

An essential component of the human diet, carbohydrates are found in many, but not all, foods. Carbohydrates often include sugars which are released when the food is digested. Many diabetics calculate their insulin doses based on the amount of carbohydrates they are about to eat. This is known as carb-counting. Carbohydrates are classified as to whether they are simple or complex carbohydrates. Usually, the more 'complex' the carbohydrate is, the slower it is to release its sugars. This forms the basis of the Glycaemic Index (GI).

DAFNE

This stands for Dose Adjustment For Normal Eating and refers to an educational programme run in the UK for people with Type 1 diabetes (who regularly blood test and inject insulin).

DESMOND

This is another education programme. The name stands for Diabetes Education and Self Management for Ongoing and Newly Diagnosed. This is aimed at people with Type 2 diabetes, explaining the nature of diabetes and looking at medications and diet.

Diabetes mellitus

This is the medical term for what is now known as Type 1 diabetes. The name more or less refers to having sugar in the blood. It is a result of not having any insulin in your body, leading to high levels of blood sugars which – untreated – can in turn result in a sugar coma.

Diabetic nephropathy

Nephropathy is kidney damage. Diabetic nephropathy is kidney damage due to high blood sugars that can result from having diabetes.

Diabetic neuropathy

Diabetic neuropathy is nerve damage due to the effects of high blood sugar which you may develop due to diabetes. It most often occurs in 'the extremities' such as hands and, in particular, feet, which is why diabetics are asked to keep an eye on their feet.

Diabetic retinopathy

Diabetic retinopathy is damage to the retina at the back of the eye due to high blood sugars that can result from having diabetes.

Frozen shoulder

This is a medical condition that anyone can get, but people with diabetes have a slightly higher incidence of having the condition than the general population. A frozen shoulder is one with restricted movement.

Gestational diabetes

A form of diabetes that occurs only during pregnancy. In the majority of women who develop gestational diabetes the condition disappears once the baby is delivered. A few patients are left still requiring medication and are therefore diabetic from that point onwards.

Glucagon, Gluco Gel, Gluco Tabs

These are brand names of sugar sources that can be used to treat a hypo. Glucagon is delivered via injection and is available on prescription. The others are fast-acting doses of sugar in either gel or tablet forms.

Glycaemic Index (GI)

A measure of how much sugar is in a food and how quickly it is released when digested.

Glycaemic Load (GL)

At most meals you will eat a combination of carbohydrates, proteins, fibre and fat. The Glycaemic Load reflects this combination so is a better indication of how food will be digested than the Glycaemic Index alone, which is based on one food in isolation.

HbA1c blood test

One of the least user-friendly medical terms around, this is the medical name for a blood sugar reading that reflects your average blood sugars over the last three months. Increasingly it is being referred to as your average BG or blood glucose.

Hyperglycaemia

The state of having a high blood sugar. Makes you feel thirsty, sluggish, tired and irritable. Needs to be treated with insulin or other diabetes medications.

Hypo dogs

This is a scheme still in its early days, but dogs have been trained to literally 'smell' a hypo and can alert their diabetic owner that they are going into a hypo. This is helpful for people who have little or no hypo warnings.

Hypoglycaemia

The state of having a low blood sugar (which is the same thing as having too much insulin in your body).

Identification tag

Depending on where you are, what you do and how stable your diabetes is, you may want to wear an identification (or I.D.) tag that states that you have diabetes. Some include which type of diabetes you have and your GP contact details. There are formats that take the form of necklaces, dog tags, bracelets or even credit card sizes, with some models specifically made for children.

Insulin

Insulin is a vital hormone which is part of a mechanism used by the body to control blood sugar levels so that, with slight variations, the levels are kept more or less stable, for example during a meal where sugars are being taken on board and digested, or during exercise where sugars (in the form of energy) are being used up. People who produce no insulin at all have diabetes mellitus (now known as Type 1 diabetes).

Short-acting or long-acting insulin – these descriptions reflect the action or release pattern of the insulin. Many patients use a combination of both to gain optimum control.

Types of insulin available:

- Analogue insulin – modern insulins that have been created to work in different ways that can fit better into some people's lives.

- Animal insulin – the original insulins were extracted from pig or cow pancreas tissue. Some are still available and some patients report that they prefer these as their release action is considered to be less harsh than the more widely available and more modern 'human' insulins.

- Human insulin – not made from humans! These are produced synthetically to emulate human insulin action.

Insulin pens

Insulin pens are one of the insulin delivery devices available. Some are made of metal, others are plastic. They can be pre-filled so insulin does not need to be loaded into them as it's already inside, or insulin cartridges can be used. Both of these types need needles to be affixed to the delivery end. Usually the insulin dose is dialled into the pen or the user counts a number of clicks, each click representing a number of insulin units being delivered. The pens are mainly produced by the insulin suppliers, with some other suppliers doing versions of pens that fit various insulin cartridges.

Insulin pump

Pumps have insulin reservoirs which are filled with just one type of insulin. They are then programmed to deliver a steady background dose of insulin (or 'basal' rate, much the same as the more familiar long-acting insulin idea) as well as doses (known as a bolus, but the same as having an injection or shot). You still need to blood test and judge your bolus and basal doses, but it's arguably more natural than five injections a day.

Islets of Langerhans

These are in the pancreas. Within the Islets of Langerhans are the alpha and beta cells. The beta cells make insulin.

Ketoacidosis (and Ketones)

In layman's terms, this is the state of going into (or being in) a sugar coma. Ketoacidosis first presents itself as a series of very high blood sugars but will progress to disorientation, loss of co-ordination and a desperate thirst. Left untreated, the patient will lose consciousness and will need hospitalisation. If your blood sugars are high, you can test for ketones. Ketones are the by-product of protein breakdown – without insulin, the body starts to break down muscle (which is protein). The patient needs insulin, nothing else will do to address this state.

Kitbag

Also known as a diabetes wallet or diabetes carry case, this is just a bag in which you can put all your diabetes kit. Having your blood test machine, medications and a sugar source to hand in case of a hypo ought to bring you some peace of mind and might help you gain and maintain good diabetes control. After diagnosis there's no need to stop doing whatever it is that you normally do, but being organised and having all your kit with you will help.

Lancets/lancing devices

I think most of us call them finger-prickers! A lancing device is used to get a drop of blood (usually from a finger) into a blood test machine in order to get a blood sugar reading.

Medical Exemption Certificate (Medex)

Thanks to the NHS, you can get your prescriptions filled for free so you do not pay for your medications. You will need a Medical Exemption Certificate to show to your pharmacist.

Pituitary gland

The pituitary gland is in the brain and helps regulate the body's internal environment. It instructs the pancreas to produce and release insulin to lower the blood sugar level if it detects that it is too high. In a person with Type 1 diabetes the pituitary still works and the messenger still gets to the pancreas, but the pancreas has no insulin to release. Hence the reason Type 1 diabetics do a blood test and use the rest of their brains to figure out what doses of insulin to give themselves.

Sharps bin

Sharps are the needles, lancets and some pump accessories that are a) sharp and b) dirty (once used). Some people would include used sensors in this category too, as they have blood on them. They should be carefully disposed of in a suitable container so that no one can accidentally prick themselves. Sharps containers are available from pharmacists. You can stick one in a kitchen cupboard and use it to put all your used bits in. When full, it should to be disposed of safely. Talk to your diabetes nurse, local GP, pharmacy or hospital about this as it varies from area to area.

Statins

These are drugs used to reduce cholesterol levels deemed to be too high. Often used in the treatment of Type 2 diabetes.

Syndrome X

Syndrome X is also known as the Metabolic Syndrome or Insulin Resistance Syndrome. It is currently being defined (by the International Diabetes Federation and American Heart Association) as a person having any three of the following: a high waist circumference indicating central obesity, high cholesterol, high blood sugar, high blood pressure and high blood sugar.

Thrush

Common enough anyway, thrush is an uncomfortable infection of the vagina (and other parts of the body) caused by a yeast called Candida. The slightly more sugary conditions in the body of someone with diabetes can lead to an increased likelihood of developing it as the yeast finds a wet, warm, sugary environment particularly handy to thrive in. It can be treated; speak to your GP or pharmacist. Good blood sugar control will reduce the risk of reoccurrence.

Traffic light system

In this system, the traffic light colours (red, amber and green) are used to help you get the balance right by helping you to choose between products and keep a check on the high-fat, high-sugar and high-salt foods you eat.

Type 1 diabetes

People who produce no insulin at all have Type 1 (once known as IDDM or Insulin-Dependent Diabetes Mellitus). It has to be treated with insulin or the patient will die. It is no longer defined just as people who take insulin and many people with Type 2 diabetes are now treated with insulin.

Type 2 diabetes

This is when people produce their own insulin but the effectiveness of that insulin is compromised. Patients can try a range of treatments to help make what insulin they do produce more effective, including diet and weight loss. Also known as insulin resistance and previously sometimes referred to as NIDDM – Non Insulin-Dependent Diabetes Mellitus.

Appendix A

Food and Blood Test Diary

FOOD NOTES   Date ...... / ...... / ......

Meal:	Time:	Result:	Food & Comments:	INSULIN:
Breakfast:				
mid-am				
Lunch:				
mid-pm				
Evening:				
late eve				

BLOOD TEST *results*

part per / mmol

These pages, designed by the author, are available as 31-day diaries from www.desang.net (0870 300 2063). Keeping notes on what you eat, when, and your dose will help you understand your diabetes better, especially if newly diagnosed or going through a rough patch. The page-to-view layout and graph system can help you track patterns – highs or lows at particular parts of your day – leading to better overall control once medications (or insulin dosage or food intake/type) are adjusted.

The shaded area on the graph highlights blood test results that fall into the 5-10 mmols/L range, rather than the more strict 4-8 mmols/L. While ALWAYS desirable, aiming to get results in the lower range can be very difficult, and a 4 is very close to a hypo, so aiming for the 5-10 mmols/L range is a bigger 'window' to aim for. Once you're regularly getting readings in that band, you can try the 'final push' to get them between 4-8 mmols/L.

Help List

General resources in the UK

There are some UK companies, websites and stores that are dedicated to diabetes supplies or who have a good range of diabetes supplies as part of their overall offering. Please note that the insulin and other diabetes medication suppliers cannot under British law liaise directly with patients about their medication. However, many do have customer care lines that can offer information about actual products (not medication) they produce as well as general information on living with diabetes. Many suppliers also have leaflets – often these are available as PDFs to download from their websites.

It is possible to buy from the USA if you buy online. You'll find a far bigger array of diabetes related goods on USA websites. However, not all of them will mail items to the UK.

Abbott Diabetes Care

Abbott House, Vanwall Business Park, Vanwall Road, Maidenhead, Berks, SL6 4UD
Tel: UK: 0500 467 466
Republic of Ireland: 1800 77 66 33
www.abbottdiabetescare.co.uk
Supplies the Precision, Optium, Freestyle, Medisense and Softsense ranges of blood test machines.

Accu-Chek brand

www.accu-chek.co.uk
Information and advice from Roche, which produces the Accu-Chek range of blood testing equipment. They also do a gestational diabetes pack as well as a diabetes and pregnancy leaflet.

Animas brand (Johnson & Johnson; Lifescan UK)

Tel: 0800 055 6606 (Animas UK & Ireland)
www.animascorp.co.uk
Newly available in the UK, Animas (linked to Lifescan UK, which produces the OneTouch Ultra blood test machines) provides insulin pumps.

Arctic Medical Ltd

Po Box 677, Folkestone, CT20 9DT
Tel: 01227 832 400
www.arcticmedical.co.uk
This site includes a comprehensive selection of products for those with diabetes, particularly injection aids.

Ascensia brand

www.ascensia.co.uk
See www.bayerdiabetes.co.uk or call Bayer Healthcare (see Bayer).
The Ascensia and Contour blood test meters are from Bayer Healthcare.

Bayer Healthcare PLC (Ascensia brand)

Bayer Healthcare, Bayer House, Strawberry Hill, Newbury, Berkshire, RG14 1JA
Tel: 0845 6006030
Diabetes Care: 01635 563 000
diabetes@bayer.co.uk
www.bayer.co.uk
Supplies the Ascensia and Contour range of blood test machines.

Bayer HealthCare (Ireland)

Bayer Ltd, The Atrium, Blackthorn Road, Dublin 18
Tel: 1 890 920111
diabetes@bayer.ie
www.bayer.ie
Supplies the Ascensia and Contour range of blood test machines.

BD Medical – Diabetes Care (Becton Dickinson UK Limited)

The Danby Building, Edmund Halley Road, Oxford Science Park, Oxford, OX4 4DQ
Tel: 01865 781 666 (customer services)
www.bdeurope.com
Suppliers of disposable syringes as well as needles for insulin pens.

The British Dietetic Association

www.bda.uk.com
The BDA is the professional association for dietitians, but their website is well worth a visit for dietary information, with a useful section called 'food facts'.

Desang Ltd

Desang Ltd, PO Box 371, Brighton, BN1 3LT
Tel: 0870 300 2063
www.desang.net
Supplies diabetes kitbags (bags designed specifically to carry both blood testing and insulin injecting diabetes management equipment), as well as other diabetes lifestyle accessories. Run by a diabetic.

Diabetes in Scotland

www.diabetes-scotland.org
This site focuses on children with Type 1 diabetes. Provides contact details for Scottish centres which care for children with diabetes.

Diabetes Research & Wellness Foundation

Tel: 023 92 637 808
www.drwf.org.uk
Provides lots of information about diabetes and how you can manage it. Includes an FAQ section and also provides leaflets. Visit their website to find out how you can become a network member and receive a copy of *Diabetes Wellness News*. Email enquiries through the website.

Diabetes UK

Tel: 0845 120 2960 (careline)

www.diabetes.org.uk

The UK's national diabetes charity for Type 1 and Type 2 diabetes. It fundraises for research purposes, publishes *Balance* magazine on a bi-monthly basis and provides a comprehensive website, with lots of information and a good list of books on diabetes. Diabetes UK is adding products to its online catalogue.

Diabeticshop.co.uk

Diabeticshop.co.uk, 184 Flanshaw Lane, Wakefield, WF2 9JD

Tel: 01924 239343 (order line)

www.diabeticshop.co.uk

A variety of diabetes products are available from this site. Run by a diabetic.

Eli Lilly and Company Limited

Lilly House, Priestley Road, Basingstoke, Hampshire, RG24 9NL

Tel: 01256 315999

www.lilly.co.uk

Supplies a range of insulins, including Humalog and Byetta, along with insulin delivery devices such as the Humapen.

Frio UK Ltd

PO Box 10, Haverfordwest, SA62 5YG

Tel: 01437 741700

info@friouk.com

www.friouk.com

Supplies a range of pouches designed to keep insulin cool and protected.

Insulin Dependent Diabetes Trust (IDDT)

PO Box 294, Northampton, NN1 4XS

www.iddtinternational.org

This group focuses on the needs of people with diabetes who are treated with insulin, particularly those who use animal-derived insulins. The website is full of information including FAQs, facts about pregnancy and diabetes and tips for living with diabetes.

Johnson & Johnson (Lifescan and Animas brands)

See Lifescan and Animas for contact details.

www.jnj.com

Supplies the Lifescan brand of blood test machines, including the One Touch and the One Touch Ultra.

Juvenile Diabetes Research Foundation (JDRF)

Juvenile Diabetes Research Foundation Head Office, 19 Angel Gate, City Road, London, EC1V 2PT

Tel: 020 7713 2030 (general enquiries)

www.jdrf.org.uk

JDRF is the only charitable organisation in the world with the primary objective of finding the cure for Type 1 diabetes and its complications.

Kids Diabetes

www.kidsdiabetes.co.uk

This colourful website is aimed at children with diabetes. Packed with information, it covers everything – from health and the body to school and recipes. Kids can sign up for a free newsletter. As the website says, adults can use it too!

Lifescan brand

www.lifescan.co.uk

Supplies the Lifescan brand of blood test machines, including the One Touch and the One Touch Ultra. Part of Johnson and Johnson.

Medic Alert

1 Bridge Wharf, 156 Caledonian Road, London, N1 9UU

Tel: 0800 581420

info@medicalert.org.uk

www.medicalert.org.uk

MedicAlert provides a life-saving identification system for individuals with hidden medical conditions and allergies. Members wear bracelets or necklets bearing the MedicAlert symbol on the disc. Each member's emblem is engraved with the wearer's main medical condition(s) and the 24-hour emergency telephone number which accepts reverse charge calls so that their specific medical details can be obtained from anywhere in the world, if necessary.

Medical Shop (Owen Mumford)

Medical Shop, Freepost OF1727, Woodstock, Oxon, OX20 1BR
Tel: 0800 731 6959 (customer careline)
www.medicalshop.co.uk
This site includes needles, sharps bins, impotence products, insulin pens (the Autolet range) and a choice of lancing devices, including the Unistic3 which is a single-use lancet.

Medicool

www.medicool.com
Although an American brand, several Medicool carry cases for diabetes can be bought in the UK from larger pharmacies and online from sites including that of Arctic Medical.

MediPAL

Communication House, 26 York Street, London, W1U 6PZ
Tel: 0845 603 4604
info@medipal.org.uk
www.medipal.org.uk
MediPAL is a plastic hard wearing card, the size of a credit card that is used as an emergency ID card or an emergency contact card. The MediPAL card shows a distinctive green cross, name / DOB, emergency contact details and 10 current medications. On the reverse of the card you can list eight important medical history details (including allergies) and your GP's name, address and telephone number or hospital contact.

Medtronic Ltd

Sherborne House, Suite One, Croxley Business Park, Watford, Herts, WD18 8WW
Tel: 01923 212213
www.medtronic-diabetes.co.uk
Supplies the Medtronic range of insulin pumps and pump accessories.

Menarini Diagnostics (Glucomen brand)

Wharfdale Road, Winnersh, Wokingham, Berkshire, RG41 5RA
Tel: 0118 9444100
www.menarinidiag.co.uk
Suppliers of the Glucomen range of blood test machines.

Novo Nordisk

Tel: 0845 600 5055 (customer care centre, Monday – Friday, 8.30am to 5.30pm.)
www.novonordisk.co.uk
Supplies the Novo range of insulins, including Novo Rapid, along with the Novopen range of insulin pens.

Roche Diagnostics Ltd (Accu-Chek brand)

See Accu-chek brand for contact details.
www.roche-diagnostics.com
Roche has the Accu-Chek range of blood test machines and the Accu-Chek Spirit insulin pump.

Sanofi-Aventis

One Onslow Street, Guildford, Surrey, GU1 4YS
Tel: 01483 505 515
www.sanofi-aventis.co.uk
Supplies Lantus insulin and insulin delivery pen.

Youth Health Talk

www.youthhealthtalk.org
This website is a collection of interviews with young people about their experiences of health or illness. The site aims to identify the issues, questions and problems that matter to young people, including diabetes.

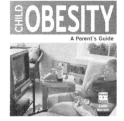 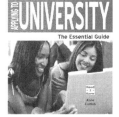 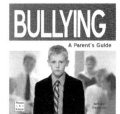 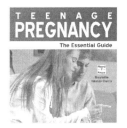 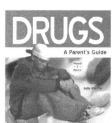